P9-DVF-784

Herpesvirus, II:
Recent Studies

A Volume in MSS' Series on Herpesvirus

Papers by
Daniel M. Albert, Jack M. Gwaltney, Jr., Joseph
H. Gainer et al.

MSS Information Corporation
655 Madison Avenue, New York, N.Y. 10021

Library of Congress Cataloging in Publication Data
Main entry under title:

Herpesvirus, I: Recent Studies

   1. Herpesvirus diseases—Addresses, essays,
lectures. 2. Herpesviruses—Addresses, essays,
lectures. I. Bellanti, Joseph A., 1934-
[DNLM: 1. Herpesvirus—Collected works. QW160.H6
H563 1973]
RC114.5.H45   616.5'2   73-13558
ISBN 0-8422-7164-3
    0-8422-7169-4 (Vol. II)
    0-8422-7176-7 (Vol. III)

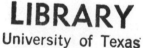

TABLE OF CONTENTS

CREDITS AND ACKNOWLEDGEMENTS

Albert, Daniel M.; and Alan S. Rabson, "Inhibition of Ocular Herpes Simplex Infection in Rabbits by Extracts of Burkitt's Lymphoma Cell Cultures," *Proceedings of the Society for Experimental Biology and Medicine*, 1971, 138:108-111.

Ashton, Heather; E. Frenk; and C.J. Stevenson, "Therapeutics. XIV. Herpes Simplex Virus Infections and Idoxuridine," *British Journal of Dermatology*, 1971, 84:496-499.

Barahana, H.H.; and L.V. Melendez, "Herpesvirus Saimiri: *In Vitro* Sensitivity to Virus-Induced Interferon and to Polyriboinosinic Acid: Polyribocytidylic Acid," *Proceedings of the Society for Experimental Biology and Medicine*, 1971, 136:1163-1167.

Docherty, John J.; Robert J. Goldberg; and Fred Rapp, "Differential Effect of 7, 12-Dimethylbenz[a]anthracene on Infectivity of Herpes Simplex Virus Type 2," *Proceedings of the Society for Experimental Biology and Medicine*, 1971, 136:328-333.

Ellery, B.W.; and D.W. Howes, "Inactivation of Infectious Laryngotracheitis Virus by Disinfectants," *Australian Veterinary Journal*, 1971, 47:330-333.

Gainer, Joseph H.; Jack Long, Jr.; Paul Hill; and Worth I. Capps, "Inactivation of the Pseudorabies Virus by Dithiothreitol," *Virology*, 1971, 45:91-100.

Gwaltney, Jack M., "Antiviral Chemotherapy," *The Virginia Medical Monthly*, 1971, 98:368-370.

Hampar, Berge; Jefferey D. Derge; Lidia M. Martos; and John L. Walker, "Persistence of a Repressed Epstein-Barr Virus Genome in Burkitt Lymphoma Cells Made Resistant to 5-Bromodeoxyuridine," *Proceedings of the National Academy of Sciences*, 1971, 68:3185-3189.

Klingeborn, B.; and Z. Dinter, "Equine Abortion (Herpes) Virus: Strain Differences in Susceptibility to Inactivation by Dithiothreitol," *Applied Microbiology*, 1972, 23:1121-1124.

Lytle, C.D., "Host-Cell Reactivation in Mammalian Cells. III. Effect of Caffeine on Herpes Virus Survival," *International Journal of Radiation Biology*, 1972, 22:167-174.

Sullivan, Robert; John T. Tierney; Edward P. Larkin; Ralston B. Read, Jr.; and James T. Peeler, "Thermal Resistance of Certain Oncogenic Viruses Suspended in Milk and Milk Products," *Applied Microbiology*, 1971, 22:315-320.

Ulbrich, A.P., "Herpes Simplex: Diagnosis and Management," *Journal of the American Osteopathic Association*, 1971, 70:1196-1198.

Underwood, G.E.; and F.R. Nichol, "Clinical Evaluation of Kethoxal Against Cutaneous Herpes Simplex," *Applied Microbiology*, 1971, 22: 588-592.

Yamamoto, Shigeru; Hidefumi Kabuta; and Yoh Nakagawa, "Inhibition of Herpes Virus Adsorption by Two Fractions Obtained from Commercial Protamine Sulfate," *The Kurume Medical Journal*, 1971, 18:39-50.

PREFACE

The Herpesviruses have an exceedingly diverse range of effects, including, as is now abundantly clear, oncogenic potentialities. This volume, part of a three-volume collection, presents papers published in 1971-1973. The research contained in this collection is intended to bring the student of the oncogenic virus up-to-date with the field.

This book, volume II, deals with modern approaches to chemotherapy of Herpesvirus infections.

Herpesvirus, I: Recent Studies, a companion volume, deals with the immunological characteristics of Herpesvirus, classification and identification of diverse Herpesvirus strains, and the relation with other diseases. Papers on Herpesvirus growth in cultured cells are also included.

Herpesvirus, III: Recent Studies, also a companion volume, presents studies on Herpesvirus effects on host cell protein synthesis and on virion phospholipid metabolism in infected cells. Additional papers dealswith nucleic acids of Herpesvirus and virus-infected cells, Herpesvirus effects on host cell chromosomes and protein components of Herpesvirus.

Inhibition of Ocular Herpes Simplex Infection in Rabbits by Extracts of Burkitt's Lymphoma Cell Cultures[1] (35841)

Daniel M. Albert and Alan S. Rabson

An inhibitor of herpes simplex virus (HSV) has been found in sonicated extracts of cell pellets of a lymphoid cell line derived from a Burkitt's lymphoma (1). The inhibitor was demonstrable in monolayer cultures of rat and human kidney cells in both plaque inhibition and 24-hr growth inhibition experiments. Although it was active against HSV, it did not significantly inhibit vesicular stomatitis virus (VSV) in similar experiments. The inhibitory activity was destroyed by boiling for 5 min, and exposure to pH 2 for 16 hr at 4°, and it was decreased fourfold by incubation with 2 mg/ml of trypsin for 1 hr at 37°. Since the lymphoma cell line produced immunoglobulins *in vitro*, the possibility that the inhibitor was an antibody to HSV was considered; however, there was no evidence of virus inactivation in a neutralization test in which virus was preincubated with the extract. On the basis of its biological properties, it was thought that the inhibitor was not interferon or an interferon inducer.

[1] This work was supported by U.S. Public Health Service grant EY-00108-02.

and the possibility that it was some type of repressor involved in the maintenance of the EB herpesvirus in a latent state in the lymphoma cells was considered.

The present studies were undertaken to determine if this inhibitor would be effective *in vivo* in the treatment of herpes simplex disease. The specific model used was herpes simplex keratitis in rabbits and the Burkitt's lymphoma extract was instilled topically into eyes infected with HSV.

Materials and Methods. The extract used was derived from AL-1 cultures of Burkitt's lymphoma, a cell line originating from a jaw tumor of a Nigerian boy (2). Cell suspensions containing 10^8 AL-1 cells/ml were obtained by low speed centrifugation and frozen at $-20°$. When suitable volumes had been collected, they were thawed and 10-ml samples were placed in a 50-ml beaker and sonicated at maximum amperage with a Branson probe sonicator for 1 min. The sonicated material was then centrifuged in a Beckman Model L ultracentrifuge with a No. 40 head for 2 hr at 30,000 rpm and the supernatant was frozen and stored in liquid nitrogen. An extract was similarly prepared from HEp-2 human epidermoid carcinoma cells (10^8 cells/ml) for use as a control.

An oral strain of HSV (No. 11124) was used to infect the corneas. The virus pool was prepared in roller bottles of HEp-2 cells and contained $10^{7.07}$ pfu/ml in a plaque assay with a methyl cellulose overlay on LBN rat kidney cells as previously described (3). Male albino New Zealand rabbits weighing 1.5 to 2 kg were used as the experimental animals. The rabbits were anesthetized with intravenous Nembutal and the right corneas were scratched with a 20-gauge needle to produce two horizontal and two vertical lines extending from limbus to limbus, each approximately 0.3 mm in depth. One-tenth ml of a suspension containing HSV (10^8 pfu) was dropped into the lower cul-de-sac of the right eye, following which the lids were manually closed and rubbed against the eye for 30 sec.

Experiments and Results. Two experiments were carried out. In the first experiment, 48 hr after the right cornea of 20 animals had been abraded and infected, the animals were divided into 10 pairs, each pair having similar appearing lesions. One animal of each pair was treated with Burkitt's lymphoma extract and the other animal served as a control. Four times daily 2 drops (approx 0.1 ml) of the Burkitt's lymphoma extract diluted 1:2 with tissue culture media (RPMI 1640 containing 20% fetal calf serum) was instilled into the lower cul-de-sac of the right eye of each treated animal and the lids were held closed for 30 sec. Treatment was continued for 7 days. Each control animal received the tissue culture media alone in a similar manner to the infected eye.

In the second experiment, treatment with Burkitt's lymphoma extract was started at 24 hr after corneal abrasion and virus infection. In addition to the control and experimental groups used in Exp. 1, there were 2 additional groups: (i) animals treated with an AL-1 extract in a dilution of 1:5; (ii) a group receiving a 1:2 dilution of an extract of HEp-2 cells that had been prepared in a manner identical to that of the Burkitt's lymphoma extract. There were 6 animals in each group. Two drops of the respective solutions were instilled into the lower cul-de-sac 4 times daily for 7 days.

Both eyes of every rabbit were examined daily with a magnifying loupe and hand light, and a slit-lamp biomicroscope both before and after the corneas were stained with fluorescein. The severity of keratoconjunctivitis thus observed was graded on a scale of 0 to 4: Grade 0 was an essentially normal appearing eye. Grade 1 constituted a well-defined epithelial lesion with slight superficial edema of the stroma limited to an area underlying the epithelial lesion; or punctate staining of the cornea. Grade 2 consisted of a more diffuse epithelial ulcer with moderate stromal edema extending beyond the epithelial defect. Grade 3 was an epithelial defect

11

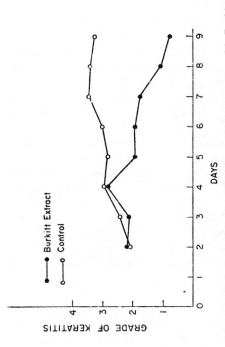

FIG. 1. Response of herpetic keratoconjunctivitis to topical treatment with Burkitt's lymphoma extract. Treatment was started 48 hr after the cornea was abraded and HSV was instilled. The control group was treated with tissue culture media alone. Grades represent the mean of 10 animals/group.

involving less than half of the corneal epithelium with severe stromal edema. Grade 4 described a defect involving more than half of the corneal epithelium with the stroma having a dense white appearance suggesting necrosis. At times ranging from 8 to 21 days after inoculation, the animals were sacrificed; and the eyes were removed and fixed in 10% buffered formalin for histopathologic study. In addition, the brains of animals with signs of encephalitis were sectioned and studied microscopically.

In the first experiment, both the treated and control groups showed an initial worsening of the keratoconjunctivitis (Fig. 1). By the fourth day of treatment, improvement was noted in the treated group while the control group continued to do poorly. Two control animals died with signs of encephalitis during the first 9 days; no treated animals were so affected.

The clinical results for the second experiment are shown in Fig. 2. Two of the control animals treated with media alone and one of the control animals receiving HEp-2 extract developed signs of encephalitis and died during the period of treatment.

Histopathologic studies of the eyes of animals treated with the Burkitt's lymphoma extract showed generally less severe or absent keratitis, uveitis, retinitis, and papillitis in the experimental eyes as compared to the control animals. Papillitis was seen in the noninfected (left) eye of the untreated animals but the optic nerve was normal in the noninfected eyes of most of the treated animals. Areas of necrosis with lymphocyte infiltration and foci of glial and vascular-endothelial proliferation were noted in the brains of animals dying of encephalitis.

Discussion. Herpetic keratitis is a major problem in clinical medicine and is the most frequent corneal infection recognizable on an etiologic or morphologic basis. The incidence and severity of the disease has been increasing and this fact has been correlated with the increasing use of topical corticosteroid hor-

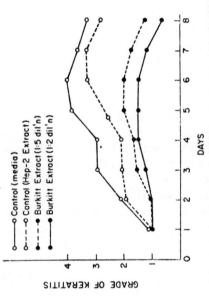
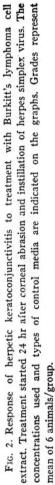

Fig. 2. Response of herpetic keratoconjunctivitis to treatment with Burkitt's lymphoma cell extract. Treatment started 24 hr after corneal abrasion and instillation of herpes simplex virus. The concentrations used and types of control media are indicated on the graphs. Grades represent mean of 6 animals/group.

mones in the eye. Discovery by Kaufman (4) that 5-iodo-2'-deoxyuridine cures or ameliorates herpes simplex keratitis has been an important advance in therapy. The response to treatment in many cases, however, remains unsatisfactory. The therapeutic use of interferon inducers such as polyI-polyC is an interesting possibility now being studied by a number of investigators (5). A soluble protein fraction has been described in the lysate of *Escherichia coli* infected by lambda-phage which inhibits intracellular replication of herpes simplex and vaccinia viruses (6, 7). Experimentally induced herpetic ulcers in the corneas of rabbits treated with this material were described as being of smaller size than those in control animals, but no clinical trials with this material have been reported.

Loss of vision due to ocular herpes infections is related to the chronic and recurrent nature of this infection. Several explanations have been offered to explain the long intervals that often occur between clinical attacks and the source of reinfection: (i) chronic asymptomatic infection of the conjunctiva and lacrimal gland has been demonstrated which could provide a source for recurring corneal infection (8); (ii) small foci of active infection have been demonstrated in corneal tissue removed during transplantation which might give rise to subsequent widespread infection (9); (iii) it has been hypothesized that herpesvirus lies dormant and undetectable in the cells of the involved tissue and becomes reactivated from this latent form (10). The presence of an inhibitor in the affected corneal cells, similar to that demonstrated in the Burkitt's lymphoma cells, could be involved in maintenance of the viral genome in a latent state.

Clarification of the chemical nature of the inhibitor and its mechanism of action will require considerable purification of the crude extracts used in these experiments. If the material can be highly purified and characterized, it is possible that it might have some therapeutic value despite the fact that it is prepared from cultures derived from neoplastic tissue. It is also possible that similar inhibitory activity might be found in extracts of lymphoid cell cultures derived from normal human lymphocytes.

Summary. Extracts of Burkitt's lymphoma cell cultures which had been previously shown to contain an inhibitor of herpes simplex virus *in vitro* were used to treat rabbits with ocular herpes infection. Topical instillation of the extract into the eyes of the rabbits cured or suppressed the progression of herpetic keratitis. Histopathologic studies of the eyes of treated and control animals confirmed the inhibition of keratitis and other evidence of herpes-related ocular inflammation.

We are grateful to Miss F. Y. Legallais, Mrs. S. A. Tyrrell and Mrs. Paula Miller for technical assistance.

1. Rabson, A. S., Tyrrell, S. A., and Legallais, F. Y., Proc. Soc. Exp. Biol. Med. 137, 264 (1971).

2. Rabson, A. S., O'Conor, G. T., Baron, S., Whang, J. J., and Legallais, F. Y., Int. J. Cancer 1, 89 (1966).

3. Rabson, A. S., Tyrrell, S. A., and Legallais, F. Y., Proc. Soc. Exp. Biol. Med. 132, 802 (1969).

4. Kaufman, H. E., Proc. Soc. Exp. Biol. Med. 109, 251 (1962).

5. Park, J. H., and Baron, S., Science 162, 811 (1968).

6. Centifanto, Y., Proc. Soc. Exp. Biol. Med. 120, 607 (1965).

7. Centifanto, Y. M., Appl. Microbiol. 16, 827 (1968).

8. Kaufman, H. E., Brown, D. C., and Ellison, E. D., Amer. J. Ophthalmol. 65, 32 (1968).

9. Hogan, M. J., Kimura, S. J., and Thygeson, P., Amer. J. Ophthalmol. 57, 551 (1964).

10. Rustigian, R., Smulow, J. B., Tye, M., Gibson, W. A., and Shindell, E., J. Invest. Dermatol. 47, 218 (1966).

Antiviral Chemotherapy

JACK M. GWALTNEY, JR., M.D.

Two chemotherapeutic agents for use in virus infections are discussed: one for treatment of herpes simplex keratitis and a second for prophylaxis against A_2 influenza.

MOST BENEFITS from antiviral drugs probably lie off in the future, and so my job as I see it today is to discuss the two currently available antiviral drugs and the three diseases in which they may have use.

The first disease which will be discussed is herpes simplex virus infection of the cornea of the eye. In some persons herpes virus is probably shed from the tear ducts or other sites for days, weeks, or even months. If a person shedding herpes virus receives a small abrasion of the cornea, this may allow the virus to attack the corneal epithelial cells and produce a typical dendritic ulcer.

17

Details of this process have recently been shown by scanning electron photomicrographs published by Spencer and Hayes from the University of California.[1] These investigators produced experimental herpes simplex ulcers on the corneas of rabbits and recorded the viral cytopathic effects which occurred in the corneal epithelial cells.

As a brief review of viral cytopathogenesis, you will recall that virus infections occur in a series of several steps. The virus is first absorbed to and then taken up by the infected cell. At this point, virus coat is removed and viral genetic material, DNA or RNA, is incorporated into the genetic information of the cell. Virus genes then control production by the infected cell of virus components which are later assembled as complete virus particles and eventually released to complete the cycle.

The antiviral drug licensed for use for herpetic keratitis is idoxuridine (IDU).* This compound is a blocking analogue of thymidine, an essential component of DNA. Success of this form of treatment depends on idoxuridine being used by the virus to form nonfunctional viral DNA. The recommended schedule of therapy is IDU ointment applied to the eye four times during the day and once during the night. Treatment is continued until the ulcer heals, usually within ten days to two weeks, and until the haze in the cornea clears which may require an additional three weeks. Thus, the total duration of therapy is usually in the range of five to six weeks.

Patients with herpes simplex keratitis may present in a way similar to that of patients

---

* Stoxil, Smith Kline & French Laboratories.

with less serious inflammations or infections of the eye. Those with minor conditions, and these patients are in the great majority, usually recover rapidly. Without proper treatment, patients with herpetic keratitis usually progress to corneal destruction. Therefore, one must consider the diagnostic problem of how to handle patients presenting with a painful and inflamed eye. I will pass on some suggestions from the experts on this, e.g., the people in the Department of Ophthalmology. They have three "don'ts" for this type of patient: (1) don't use topical steroids alone or in combination with other drugs; (2) don't use preparations containing local anesthetic agents; (3) don't use the ointment form of drugs. (The one exception being IDU ointment which is preferred over IDU solution.) The contraindicated forms of treatment, although usually successful with minor cases of eye inflammation, tend to make herpes virus infections worse. Patients on topical steroids or anesthetics may have subjective improvement while the ulcer progresses to a perforation of the cornea. Prior use of steroid therapy and ointments may also delay healing at the time specific antiviral therapy is started. Both topical steroids and ointments tend to interfere with the appearance of new corneal epithelial cells at the ulcer site of IDU treated patients.

As substitutes for these preparations, the ophthalmologists recommend sulfacetamide, 10% solution*, or a combination of topical antibiotics such as polymyxin, neomycin, and gramicidin solution**. Patients who

---

* Sulamyd—White Laboratories.
** Neosporin—Burroughs Wellcome Company.

19

do not recover in a week to ten days on one of these preparations and cold soaks should be evaluated for herpes virus or fungus infection of the cornea.

The diagnosis of herpes virus infection of the eye has been made in the past on the characteristic appearance of the dendritic ulcer. It is now easy to isolate herpes virus in a laboratory using one of several commercially available tissue cultures such as human embryonic lung cells, WI-38. Tissue culture methods are becoming more widely used and are currently available in the State Laboratory in Richmond.

The second disease which will be discussed is herpes virus encephalitis. This form of encephalitis is the most common of the severe life threatening forms of encephalitis recognized in Virginia today. Herpes encephalitis may be more common than has been recognized because it is virtually impossible to establish the diagnosis without a brain biopsy. Biopsy is done to obtain material for virus culture and pathologic examination. Herpes simplex infection should be suspected in all cases of severe encephalitis. This disease may have an intermittent course over days or weeks, and acute psychotic episodes have been described as one of its manifestations. Herpes virus encephalitis usually presents a different picture from the more common cases of enterovirus meningitis. Most patients with the latter disease are essentially well within two to four days.

There is some suggestion from isolated case reports and a small series[2] that intravenous IDU may be beneficial and even life saving in patients with herpes simplex encephalitis. If IDU therapy is effective, it seems reasonable that it should be given early at a time before severe and irreversible neurologic damage has occurred. For this reason, the diagnosis must be suspected early in the course of the illness. Unfortunately, we are often called to see patients late in the course of encephalitis after their condition has become hopeless, at which time we are reluctant to recommend brain biopsies. It should also be pointed out that intravenous IDU has serious toxic side effects and that treatment of herpes encephalitis with this drug is still considered an experimental procedure.

The last drug I will discuss is amantadine*. The antiviral action of this compound is to prevent the penetration of virus particles into the cell. Amantadine is active against the A strains of influenza virus, including the Hong Kong strain, but, curiously, it is not active against influenza type B. At the present time, amantadine is licensed only for prophylactic use against Asian A_2 influenza. Since Asian strains have been replaced in the population by the Hong Kong strains of virus, amantadine has become legally obsolete.

More recently trials have been carried out to determine if amantadine has a therapeutic effect against A_2 influenza. Data from a study done in Richmond by Dr. Wingfield et al.[3] show the type of evidence available on this question. Patients with natural influenza virus infection treated with amantadine showed more rapid clinical improvement as determined by an index of

---

* Symmetrel, DuPont de Nemours & Company.

illness severity than did patients on placebo. Also, patients on amantadine became afebrile in a shorter period of time than did those on placebo. Similar results have been obtained in other studies including one by Dr. Knight et al. at Baylor[4] in which it was also shown that the amount of virus shed by volunteers on the drug was less than that shed by persons on placebo. Thus, amantadine appeared to actually lessen the amount of virus infection that occurred in treated subjects. It remains to be seen if, by inhibiting virus multiplication, amantadine can prevent or retard the serious and sometimes fatal complication of virus pneumonia. The answer to this question is obviously important in an assessment of the therapeutic value of amantadine.

Summary

Two antiviral compounds are available for clinical use. Idoxuridine has proven to be effective in the treatment of herpes simplex keratitis. For maximum benefit from this compound, patients should not receive previous treatment with steroids, local anesthetics, or ointments. IDU may also be beneficial, if given early, to patients with herpes encephalitis, but this must be regarded as an experimental form of therapy. A second antiviral agent, amantadine, has prophylactic and, to a moderate degree, therapeutic action against A_2 influenza. Strains of the currently circulating Hong Kong virus are sensitive to the drug, however, it has not received FDA approval for use against these new viruses. Also, amantadine is not approved for therapeutic use at present. An important unanswered question about this compound is, will it prevent the serious complication of influenza pneumonia?

REFERENCES

1. Spencer, W. H. and Hayes, T. L.: Scanning and Transmission Electron Microscope Observations of the Topographic Anatomy of Dendritic Lesions in the Rabbit Cornea. Invest. Ophth. 9:183-195, 1970.
2. Nolan, D. C., Carruthers, M. M., and Lerner, A. M.: Herpesvirus Hominis Encephalitis in Michigan. Report of Thirteen Cases, Including Six Treated with Idoxuridine. New England J. M. 282:10-13, 1970.
3. Wingfield, W. L., Pollack, D., and Grunert, R. R.: Therapeutic Efficacy of Amantadine HCl and Rimantadine HCl in Naturally Occurring Influenza A_2 Respiratory Illness in Man. New England J. M. 281:579-584, 1969.
4. Knight, V., Fedson, D., Baldini, J., Douglas, R. G., and Couch, R. B.: Amantadine Therapy of Epidemic Influenza A_2 (Hong Kong). Inf. & Immun. 1:200-204, 1970.

ACKNOWLEDGMENT:

I would like to express my appreciation to Dr. Ellison Conrad of the Department of Ophthalmology, University of Virginia Hospital, for his advice on the diagnosis and management of patients with herpetic keratitis and other infections of the eye.

Presented at the annual meeting of The Medical Society of Virginia, Richmond, October 11-14, 1970.

Inactivation of the Pseudorabies Virus by Dithiothreitol

JOSEPH H. GAINER, JACK LONG, JR.,

PAUL HILL, AND WORTH I. CAPPS

The virucidal nature of reduced dithiothreitol (DTT) for the pseudorabies (PR) virus (PRV) is presented. The rate of decay of PRV in DTT increased exponentially as the pH rose from 6.5 to 8. Effective virucidal concentrations of DTT decreased in concentration as the pH was elevated. The reaction rate was temperature dependent under mild alkaline conditions, being essentially nil at $0°$ and at $20°$, but progressively more rapid from $30°$ to $41°$. Electron micrographs indicated substantial disruption of the architecture of the DTT inactivated virions.

Preincubation of DTT with catalytic amounts of Cu^{2+} or with high concentrations of Mg^{2+} decreased the virucidal activity; preincubation with catalytic levels of Fe^{3+} lowered activity slightly.

Thirteen additional compounds, mostly thiols, were tested for virucidal activities. Reduced dithioerythritol (DTE), an asymmetric isomer of DTT, was considerably less active than DTT. British anti-lewisite (BAL), (2,3-dimercapto-1-propanol), was of the same order of activity as DTE, but 1,3-dimercapto-2-propanol, an isomer of BAL, was essentially nonvirucidal. Thimerosal and iodoacetamide at 0.01 M were virucidal, but 2-mercaptoethanol at 0.01 M was inactive. Trithiodiglycol at 0.01 M, pH 8.0, was moderately virucidal. Oxidized dithiothreitol was nonvirucidal.

INTRODUCTION

Reduced dithiothreitol, a sluggish disulfide bond-reducing agent (Cleland, 1964), has been shown to inactivate members of the arbovirus groups A and B, the poxvirus vaccinia, and the myxovirus Newcastle disease; on the other hand, it was not virucidal for three enteroviruses tested—Coxsackie B₅ , polio type 2, and echo 6 (Carver and Seto, 1968). It has been shown to possess slight virucidal activity against polyoma virus at high pH (Hare and Chan, 1968). DTT has not been reported as a virucide against any herpesvirus.

This paper illustrates that DTT rapidly inactivates PRV under limiting conditions of temperature, pH, and drug concentration. The results of these experiments and others, describing conditions or limitations of the inactivation process, are presented. Related monothiols, dithiols, one trithiol, and several other compounds presumed to be virucidal because of a similar mechanism of action to DTT were tested.

Chemicals. Oxidized and reduced dithiothreitol, oxidized and reduced glutathione, and DL-cysteine were purchased from Calbiochem. Corp., Los Angeles, California. Reduced dithioerythritol was purchased from Nutritional Biochemicals, Cleveland, Ohio. Other compounds were purchased from commerically available sources as listed in Table 3.

Virus and tissue cultures. PRV was pre-prepared in primary rabbit kidney (PRK) cells (Grand Island Biological Co., Grand Island, New York), or in continuous line rabbit kidney (RK-13) cells (Flow Laboratories, Rockville, Maryland) propagated in our laboratory. Tissue culture medium was modified McCoy's 5A containing 10% fetal calf serum and penicillin, streptomycin, and fungizone. Several pools of virus were prepared by inoculating fully sheeted PRK monolayers with a 10^{-2} dilution of PRV (2 PFU/cell). Plastic tissue culture bottles, 75 cm² (Falcon Plastic, Becton-Dickinson, Baltimore, Maryland) were used. Virus was in its 15th to 20th passage. The strain of PRV was isolated in Florida from the lymph node of a pig dying with signs of pseudorabies infection. Proved identity of the isolate was made by neutralization of the virus with specific PRV antiserum supplied us from the National Animal Disease Laboratory, Ames, Iowa. Unpurified virus (PRV-U) was harvested when 90% of the cells had undergone advanced cytopathology, 24 hours after inoculation. The infected material was frozen and thawed 3 times, centrifuged at 2000 rpm for 20 min at 4°, and the supernatant was decanted and saved. The pellets were sonicated momentarily with a sonicator (Branson Sonifer Cell Disrupter, Heat Systems Co., Melville, Long Island, New York) in minimum spent culture medium. The spent medium was returned to the sonicate, clarified by low speed centrifugation, distributed into 1 ml, or larger quantities, and stored at −80°.

Partially purified virus (PRV-P) was prepared by centrifuging the PRV-U 40,000 rpm for 1 hr at 5°. Pellets were rinsed momentarily with 0.85% NaCl solution, resuspended in $\frac{1}{5}$ to $\frac{1}{10}$ the original volume in 0.85% NaCl, distributed in 0.6 ml or larger quantities, and stored at −80°.

Procedure. Drugs were prepared freshly each day, the thiols being dissolved in sterile distilled water until time arrived for the preparation of specific mixtures. Drug, drug-virus, or virus dilution were maintained at 0° until experiments were begun. Tissue cultures for assays were confluent monolayers of 7–10-day PRK cells or RK-13 cells cultivated in Falcon 15 × 60 mm dishes, incubated at 37° in 5% CO_2. Virus, 0.4 ml, was permitted to adsorb to the cells for 90 min, at 37°, with gentle rotation of the plates at 15–20-min intervals. In decay studies, reaction mixtures were performed/prepared in plastic or glass tubes or glass vials—all of the same kind of container within each experiment. Reaction mixtures were chilled in ice-water to stop the reactions before dilutions for assays were made. Unless indicated otherwise, virus-drug mixtures were prepared in Earle's balanced salt solution (EBSS) and incubated at 37°. Following adsorption of virus, 6 ml of agar overlay, consisting of medium 199, 5% fetal calf serum, and 0.7% Ionagar, plus antibiotics, was added per plate. Plates were incubated 1 day at 37°; they were stained with 2 ml of medium 199 agar overlay, containing 1:20,000 neutral red. Plaques were counted after 24 hr additional incubation.

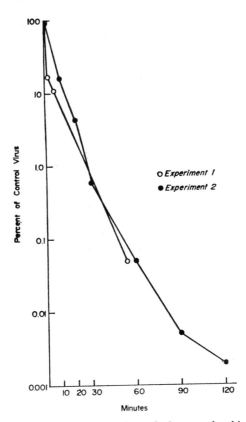

FIG. 1. The inactivation of the pseudorabies virus by dithiothreitol. PRV-U, 10^7 PFU, was incubated in 0.002 M DTT for 54 min, (experiment 1) or 120 min (experiment 2). Aliquots were removed at indicated times and chilled. Reaction mixtures and dilutions were made in EMEM containing 1% serum. The 54-min study was assayed on PRK cells, the 120-min study, in RK-13 monolayers.

RESULTS

The Effect of Variations in Temperature, pH, and Several Components on the Rate of Inactivation of PRV by DTT; Electron Microscopy

PRV was first tested with DTT in Eagle's Minimal Essential Medium EM-EM) (Fig. 1). Rapid inactivation of virus followed.

Figure 2 illustrates the relative rates of decay of PRV in DTT at various tempera-

27

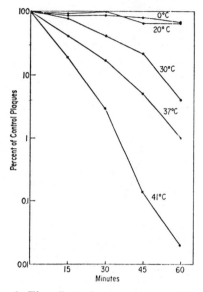

Fig. 2. The effect of temperature on the pseudorabies virucidal activity of dithiothreitol. DTT, 0.001 M, was incubated with 7×10^6 PFU of PRV-U in 0.05 M phosphate —NaOH buffer, pH 7.5, containing 1% serum. At times indicated, aliquots were diluted 1:10 in cold buffer to stop further action. Assays were made in PRK cells.

tures. It is noted that at 0° and 20° little inactivation occurred. However, at 30° and above, the rate of inactivation increased as the temperature rose.

Table 1 illustrates a substantial reduction in the virucidal activity of DTT when it was incubated with high levels of Mg^{2+} prior to the addition of virus. It is noted that the presence of Mg^{2+} in control plates stimulated PFU numbers. It is assumed that the reduction in effect is through the chelating action of DTT for the magnesium, the Mg^{2+} being chelated by the SH groups of the DTT so that the DTT is no longer capable of reducing (inactivating) the virus. Cleland (1964) stated that DTT in solution forms a ring structure, the H atoms being lost from the SH groups during reduction, and metals being readily chelatable at the open end of the claw. Oxidized glutathione (OGSH), when incorporated in the DTT-PRV mixture in equimolar concentrations with DTT,

28

TABLE 1

THE REDUCTION IN VIRUCIDAL ACTIVITY OF DITHIOTHREITOL BY PRIOR INCUBATION WITH MAGNESIUM[a]

Concentration of MgSO$_4$	Residual virus (% of control)	Number of plaques in controls at $10^{-4.6}$ dilution of PRV
0.02 M	17	63
0.002 M	12	42
None	1[b]	32

[a] Procedure: DTT, 0.002 M was incubated with 0.02 M MgSO$_4$, 0.002 M MgSO$_4$, or distilled water for 10 min at 37°. Solutions were iced; PRV-P, 1 × 10^6 PFU, was added and adjusted to pH 8.0 with boric acid buffer, 0.05 M; incubation was permitted for an additional 10 min at 37°. Virus controls were incubated in MgSO$_4$ solutions and diluted in boric acid buffer without any DTT. Platings were made on RK-13 cells. Final DTT concentration in the presence of virus was 0.001 M.

[b] This is a conservative maximum estimate based upon another similar experiment (Fig. 5); the titration end point was not reached in this trial.

TABLE 2

THE EFFECT OF OXIDIZED GLUTATHIONE, DITHIOTHREITOL, AND MIXTURES THEREOF ON THE INACTIVATION OF PSEUDORABIES VIRUS

Drug	Final drug concentration	Percent of control virus
Dithiothreitol, reduced	0.003 M	0.02
Oxidized Glutathione	0.003 M	64.2
Both	0.003 M each	76.0

[a] An equal volume of DTT, oxidized GSH, or mixtures thereof was added to 2 × 10^6 PFU of PRV-U in EMEM. They were incubated for 1 hr and plated on PRK cells.

abolished all viral inactivation (Table 2). OGSH presumably oxidizes the reduced DTT at a more rapid rate than what the virus does, the OGSH competing with virus

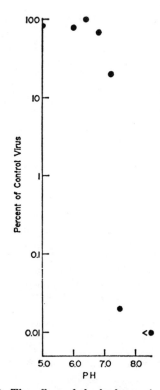

FIG. 3. The effect of the hydrogen ion concentration on the pseudorabies virucidal activity of dithiothreitol. This figure represents several experiments. Final DTT concentrations of 0.0008 M were incubated for 1 hr with 2 lots of PRV-P at various pHs indicated. One lot of virus contained 2.5×10^4 PFU, the other contained 16×10^6 PFU. Buffers were 0.05 M with respect to the first component of various mixtures as follows: (1) pH 3.0 to 6.2 were phthalate-NaOH mixtures; (2) pH 5.8 to 8.0 were KH_2PO_4–NaOH mixtures; and, (3) pH 7.8 to 10.0 were boric acid–NaOH mixtures. There was slight decay (up to 50%) of virus in controls in the pH range of 5.0 to 8.0 after 1 hr; above pH 8.0, the virus decayed rapidly. Assays were made in RK-13 monolayers. The large difference in titers of the 2 virus pools did not materially affect the results.

for reduction by DTT.

Several experiments were conducted to determine the effect of pH on the PR virucidal activity of DTT. Figure 3 illustrates such effects when a 0.0008M final drug

30

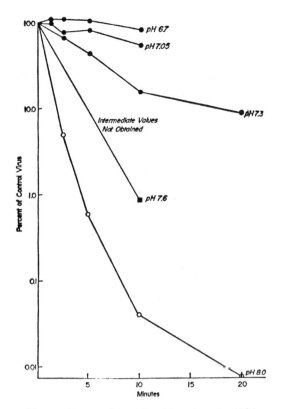

FIG. 4. Decay of pseudorabies virus in dithiothreitol at various hydrogen ion concentrations. This figure represents 2 experiments, both employing 0.002 M DTT. PRV-P, 1.5×10^4 PFU, was incubated for various times with DTT at pH 6.7, 7.1 and 7.5, the beginning pHs. The pHs, redetermined after 10 min incubation, were 6.7, 7.05, and 7.6, as stated in the figure. In the second experiment, PRV-P, 4×10^6 PFU, was tested in DTT at pH 7.3 or pH 8.0. KH$_2$PO$_4$–NaOH buffer, 0.05 M, was used throughout; assays were made in RK-13 cells.

concentration was tested. Figure 4 illustrates the kinetics of decay at various pHs in 0.002 M DTT. Figure 5 illustrates the decay rate of PRV in various concentrations of DTT at pH 7.3 and at pH 8.0. It is noted in these experiments the strong dependence of virucidal action of DTT on pH.

Data from several experiments were summarized to illustrate the time required for the first 50% decay (T/50) of PRV at

31

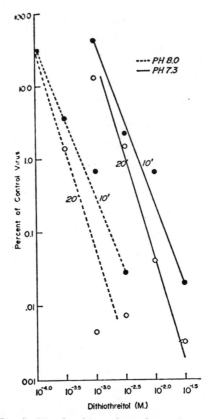

FIG. 5. Pseudorabies virus decay in various concentrations of dithiothreitol at pH 7.3 and at pH 8.0. PRV-P, 5×10^6 PFU, was incubated for 10 or 20 min with varying concentrations of DTT at pH 7.3 or pH 8.0, in 0.05 M KH$_2$PO$_4$–NaOH buffer. Assays were made in RK-13 monolayers.

various pHs (Fig. 6). A sigmoid type of curve is noted with activity being pH dependent between 6.5 and 8.0. Outside these pH ranges the curve flattened out. Above pH 8.0, the strong base itself rapidly inactivated the virus so that the kinetics of inactivation of PRV by DTT in a strong base was not determinable; from pH 6.5 to 5.0, no essential differences in effect occurred.

Figure 7 illustrates the physical appearance of DTT treated virus compared to untreated virus. The treated virions are distorted; they have lost their internal architecture and they have taken up more

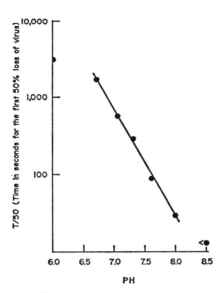

FIG. 6. Time required for 50% decay ($T/50$) of pseudorabies virus in dithiothreitol at various hydrogen ion concentrations. This figure was extrapolated from several other experiments wherein the time in seconds for the first 50% loss of virus in DTT was determined. Several lots of PRV-P were used with titers ranging from $10^{4.5}$ to 10^7 PFU/ml. Reactions were performed in 0.002 M DTT. Buffer mixtures were 0.05 M as stated in Fig. 3. Although the pools of virus varied considerably in titer, variations in these titers did not influence the results to any appreciable extent.

of the strain than have the untreated particles.

Comparisons of Compounds Similar to DTT for Virucidal Capabilities

Figure 8 compares the PR vircuidal effects of DTT with DTE. Figure 9 illustrates the structural formulas of 4 dithiols and their relative potencies as PR virucides. One notes a 50,000-fold difference in magnitude of action between the most active compound and the least active compound.

Table 3 compares several dithiols, a monothiol, one trithiol, and several other compounds for PR virucidal activity.

Catalytic amounts of $FeCl_3$ and $CuCl_2$ have been shown (Barron *et al.*, 1947) to oxidize reduced dithiols rapidly, $CuCl_2$ being

33

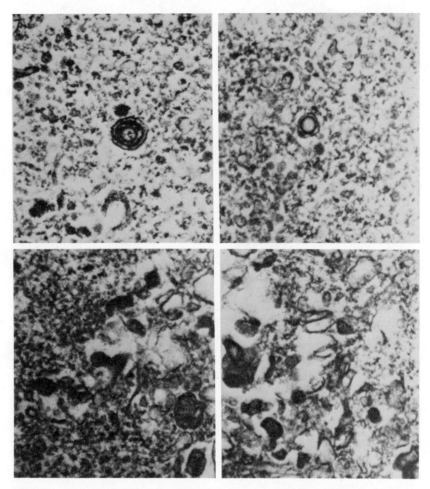

FIG. 7. Electron micrographs of pseudorabies virus untreated and treated with dithiothreitol. PRV-P, 1.4 × 10⁸ PFU, was incubated in 0.05 M pH 8.0 KH₂PO₄–NaOH buffer with 0.002 M DTT for 30 min; untreated virus was incubated in pH 8.0 buffer without DTT. Samples were chilled to 5° and centrifuged at 40,000 rpm for 1 hr. Pellets were fixed in 4% glutaraldehyde, postfixed in osmium tetroxide, embedded in Epon, sectioned, stained with uranyl acetate–lead nitrate, and examined in a Phillip's 300 electron microscope. The upper prints contain 1 each untreated PRV virion; the lower prints contain many distorted and heavily stained DTT treated virions. × 49,756.

TABLE 3

STUDIES OF MICELLANEOUS COMPOUNDS FOR PSEUDORABIES VIRUCIDAL ACTIVITY[a]

Name of compound	Source of compound	Final concentration of compound (M)	Reactions in	
			EMEM or in EBSS ph 7.3–7.6	Boric acid buffer, 0.05 M pH 8.0
1. 2-Thiobarbituric acid	Calbiochem., Los Angeles, Calif.	0.01	49[b]	59
2. Dithiodiglycolic acid	Aldrich Chem., Milwaukee, Wisc.	0.01	34	39
3. 2-Hydroxyethyl disulfide	Aldrich Chem., Milwaukee, Wisc.	0.01	50	85
4. 1,3-Dimercapto-2-propanol	Aldrich Chem., Milwaukee, Wisc.	0.01	33	62
5. 2,2-Dithio-bis-(ethylamine)2-2-HCl	Calbiochem., Los Angeles, Calif.	0.01	36	87
6. Trithiodiglycol	K&K Laboratories, Plainview, New York	0.01·	24	10
7. N-Ethyl maleimide	K&K Laboratories, Plainview, New York	0.01	4.3	ND[c]
		0.001	67	ND
8. 2,3-Dimercapto-1-propanol	J. T. Baker Chem. Co., Phillipsburg, N. J.	0.01	0.1[d]	ND
9. Thimerosal	Nutritional Biochem., Cleveland, Ohio	0.01	0.2[d]	0.3
		0.001	90[d]	ND
		0.0004	98[d]	ND
10. Iodoacetamide	K&K Laboratories, Plainveiw, New York	0.01	2.4[d]	0.0
		0.001	29[d]	ND
		0.0004	28[d]	ND
11. 2-Mercaptoethanol	Eastman-Kodak Co., Rochester, New York	0.01	125[d]	57
		0.0004	100[d]	ND
12. DL-Cysteine	Calbiochem., Los Angeles, Calif.	0.01	110[d]	100
		0.001	94[d]	ND
		0.0004	74[d]	ND

[a] Drug and virus, 2.5×10^6 PFU of PRV-U, were mixed and incubated for 1 hr. Assays were made in either RK-13 or PRK cells.

[b] Results are expressed as percent of virus control plaques.

[c] ND, not done.

[d] Reactions in EMEM; all others in EBSS in this column.

a much more rapid oxidizer than $FeCl_3$; other metal salts tested—Mg^{2+}, Co^{2+}, and Mn^{2+}—had no effects. Ferric chloride, $MgCl_2$, and $CuCl_2$ were tested as catalysts for the abolishment of the virucidal activity of DTT by incubation with DTT prior to adding virus (Table 4). Cupric chloride abolished to a substantial extent the virucidal activity of DTT; $FeCl_3$ had a slight effect, and $MgCl_2$ was nonreactive.

DISCUSSION

Results of these experiments illustrate that reduced DTT readily inactivates PRV under appropriate conditions of temperature and pH. The first 50% decay of virus in DTT followed an exponential rate as the pH was increased from 6.5 to 8.0.

Preincubation of DTT with high levels of magnesium, 0.01 M, accounted for reduced virucidal activity, presumably because the DTT chelated the Mg and less DTT was therefore available for virucidal action.

The decay rate was seemingly more dependent upon the concentration of DTT than on concentration of virus. Note the extent of inactivation compared with DTT concentration in Fig. 5; on the other hand, essentially the same amount of inactivation followed over the same time and same DTT concentration in Fig. 4 and Fig. 5, even though virus concentration varied 100-fold. The presence or absence of 1% serum in reaction mixtures did not affect results: compare Figs. 2 and 8, which had it with Figs. 3, 4, and 5, which did not.

It is estimated, by rough approximations, that at pH 7.3 or slightly higher on the order of 10^9 to 10^{10} molecules of DTT must be present per PFU of PRV before viral decay may proceed. The concentration of DTT necessary for virucidal action fell inversely in essentially the same proportions as the pH increased. It is noted that $\frac{1}{10}$ the concentration of drug was needed to account for the same amount of virus decay when the reaction was performed at

TABLE 4

The Reduction in Virucidal Activity of
Dithiothreitol When Preincubated with
Catalytic Amounts of Various Metals[a]

	Infective virus, percent of each metal control	Relative percent residual virucidal activity of DTT
$CuCl_2 \cdot 2H_2O$	54%	46
$FeCl_3 \cdot 6H_2O$	3%	97
$MgCl_2 \cdot 6H_2O$	0.6%	99.4
DTT Controls without Metal Salt Added	1.2%	98.8

[a] Respective metal salts at 0.00004 M were incubated with DTT, 0.002 M for 10 min at 37°. The reaction mixtures were chilled, and 1×10^6 PFU of PRV-P was added; reincubation was permitted for 10 min, 37°. Assays were made on RK-13 cells.

pH 8.0 as at pH 7.3. This 10-fold increase in magnitude of vircuidal activity approximates the 15-fold increase in equilibrium constant for the conversion of DPN+ to DPNH by DTT as the pH is increased from 7.0 to 8.1 (Cleland, 1964). The higher pH is accounting for a more rapid decay rate.

Dithioerythritol (DTE), an asymmetric isomer of DTT, was about $\frac{1}{10}$ as virucidal as DTT. The lesser activity of DTE compared to DTT may be through its asymmetric nature, through this asymmetry, it just cannot collide as efficiently with virus as can DTT.

When 2,3-dimercapto-1-propanol (BAL) was compared with its isomer, 1,3-dimercapto-2-propanol, a large difference in magnitude of effect was noted—BAL was of essentially the same order of vircuidal activity as was DTE, but the 1,3 isomer of BAL was essentially nonvirucidal. The physical arrangement of the 1,3 isomer presumably prevents its ready reaction with PRV in contrast to the 2,3 isomer.

Oxidized glutathione (OGSH) inhibited the PR virucidal activity of DTT, presumably because OGSH can readily and spe-

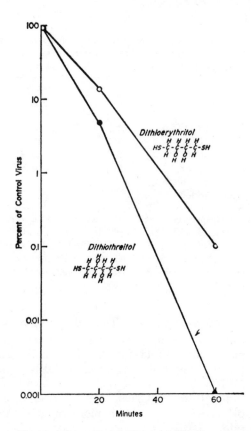

Fig. 8. The comparative pseudorabies virucidal activities of dithiothreitol and dithioerythritol. PRV-U, 1.2×10^7 PFU, was incubated with
0.002 M drugs, for 20 min or 60 min; 1% fetal calf
serum was present in the reaction mixtures. Both
drugs were in the reduced state. Following incubation, samples were plated on PRK cells. Included
in the experiment was a trail with 0.002 M oxidized
DTT; it was essentially nonvirucidal in that
86 and 95% remaining virus was present following
20 min and 60 min incubation, respectively.

cifically oxidize DTT. It appears on the other
hand that any oxidizing agent will oxidize
DTT. In the experiment in which $CuCl_2$,
$FeCl_3$, and $MgCl_2$ were tested for their
ability to oxidize DTT, it is noted that
$CuCl_2$ in catalytic amounts readily inhibited the virucidal activity of DTT,
presumably through oxidation. Of these 3
compounds, $CuCl_2$ was the best oxidizing

RELATIVE PSEUDORABIES VIRUCIDAL ACTIVITIES OF CLOSELY RELATED DITHIOLS

NAME	STRUCTURE	PSEUDORABIES VIRUS DECAY IN DRUG 37C 1HR	MAGNITUDE OF DIFFERENCE
Dithiothreitol (DTT)	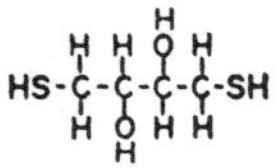 HS-C-C-C-C-SH	0.001[a]	100 Fold
Dithioerythritol (DTE)	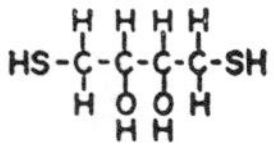 HS-C-C-C-C-SH	0.1	
2,3-Dimercapto-1-propanol (BAL)	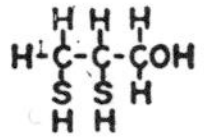 H-C-C-C-OH	0.1	500 Fold
1,3-Dimercapto-2-propanol	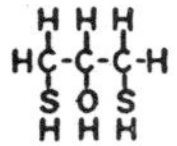 H-C-C-C-H	50	

[a]*Percent of Control Virus Remaining*

FIG. 9. Comparative pseudorabies virucidal activities of four dithiols. PRV-U, 10^6 PFUs, was incubated with each of the 4 dithiols listed for 1 hr. BAL and 1,3-dimercapto-2-propanol were final concentrations of 0.005 M; DTT and DTE were final concentrations of 0.002 M. Samples were assayed in PRK cells.

39

salt. Catalytic levels of $MgCl_2$ were inactive, in contrast to activity of Mg^{2+} when a 40 to 400 times more concentrated solution was tested. $CuCl_2$, when tested alone with virus and in combination with DTT and virus to learn if it reacted like OGSH as a reverser of DTT, was found to be PR virucidal itself.

Oxidized DTT was nonvirucidal. Of the several miscellaneous compounds tested, it is surprising that 2-mercaptoethanol was not virucidal; it is possible that it was not in the reduced state when tested, or it may be virucidal for PRV only at higher concentrations.

These studies indicate that the protein coat of the pseudorabies virion reacts readily, presumably through reduction, by the reducing agent dithiothreitol. The electron micrographs indicate a marked alteration in the physical appearance and stainability of the virion following treatment with DTT. It is proposed that the DTT is disrupting and apparently cleaving the protein coat of the virion at the cystine S-S linkages. Hare and Chan, 1968, have shown by electron microscopy that treatment of polyoma virus with DTT in strong base disrupts that virus.

This paper adds an encapsulated virus of the herpesvirus group to the list of encapsulated viruses (Carver and Seto, 1967) which can be inactivated by the disulfide bond reducing agent DTT. It does not clarify the paper (Phillipson and Choppin, 1962) wherein nonencapsulated enteroviruses were inactivated by BAL, and reportedly more efficiently by oxidized BAL than by reduced BAL. In this study, BAL, presumably in the reduced state, was found considerably less reactive than DTT for inactivation of PRV.

Finally, these studies illustrate the necessity, especially in drug screening programs, to vary the pH, the temperature, and other components of reaction mixtures before it is possible to state whether a compound is virucidal or not.

ACKNOWLEDGMENT

The authors thank the Pathologic Anatomy Branch of our Institute for their preparation of the electron micrographs. The senior author gratefully acknowledges and sincerely thanks Dr. John W. Needham, Chemical Abstracts, Columbus, Ohio, for helpful advice during the course of this study.

REFERENCES

BARRON, E. S. G., MILLER, Z. B., and KALNITSKY, G. (1947). The oxidation of dithiols. *Biochem. J.* **41**, 62-68.

CARVER, D. H., and SETO, D. S. Y. (1968). Viral inactivation by disulfide bond reducing agents. *J. Virol.* **2**, 1482-1484.

CLELAND, W. W. (1964). Dithiothreitol, a new protective reagent for SH groups. *Biochemistry* **3**, 480-482.

HARE, J. D., and CHAN, J. C. (1968). Role of hydrogen and disulfide bonds in polyoma capsid structure. *Virology* **34**, 481-491.

PHILLIPSON, L., and CHOPPIN, P. W. (1962). Inactivation of enteroviruses by 2,3-dimercaptopropanol (BAL). *Virology* **16**, 405-413.

Equine Abortion (Herpes) Virus: Strain Differences in Susceptibility to Inactivation by Dithiothreitol

B. KLINGEBORN AND Z. DINTER

The infectivity of equine abortion (herpes) virus (EAV) was inactivated by treatment with reduced dithiothreitol (DTT). According to their susceptibility to DTT, the EAV strains could be divided into three groups. The vaccine strain RAC-H (419) proved to be more resistant to DTT than all of the other 14 strains tested. The hemagglutinin of EAV was also inactivated by DTT; no strain differences were observed in this respect.

Reduced dithiothreitol (DTT) is a slow acting agent which reduces disulfide bonds. It was first described by Cleland (3). Several viruses have been shown to be inactivated by DTT. Among these viruses are members of the arbovirus groups A and B, the poxvirus vaccinia, the paramyxovirus Newcastle disease (2), and the papovavirus polyoma (7). A herpesvirus, the pseudorabies virus, has been reported to be inactivated by DTT under limiting conditions of temperature, pH, and drug concentration (6). Other viruses which have been tested, i.e., some picornaviruses, proved to be resistant to inactivation by DTT (2).

In the present report, the inactivation by DTT of another herpesvirus, the equine abortion virus (EAV), is described. However, various EAV strains showed differences in sensitivity to DTT, the vaccine strain RAC-H (8) being the most resistant one. This strain is also characterized by its inability to produce plaques in L cells (1).

MATERIALS AND METHODS

Cell cultures. Four different types of cells were used: PK-15, a continuous line of pig kidney cells; KFBL, a line of bovine lung cells transformed by simian virus 40 deoxyribonucleic acid (4); and two different clones of L cells. One clone (L-B) was supplied by H. C. Borgen, Lindholm, Denmark, and the other one (L-929) was obtained from Flow Laboratories, Irvine, Scotland. Eagle's minimal essential medium (MEM) with 5% calf serum (KFBL) or MEM without serum (PK-15, L-929) was used for maintenance. The medium for the L-B cells and the methylcellulose overlay for both L-cell clones were those recommended by Borgen (1).

EAV strains. Fifteen different EAV strains were used. Two of them were derivatives of the hamster-adapted RAC-H strain which was passaged in pig kidney cells (8). We obtained the low-passage RAC-H strain, referred to as 17, and the high-passage RAC-H strain (the vaccine strain), referred to as 419, by courtesy of A. Mayr, Munich, Germany. Strains N-3 and SL-D were kindly supplied by H.C. Borgen. The 11 other strains used were low-passage isolates derived from aborted fetuses. Stock virus of each strain was harvested as culture fluid from infected PK-15 cells and stored at -60 C. Purified virus preparations of strains 419 and 647 had also been used. The purification procedure was described elsewhere (7a).

End-point titrations. End-point titrations were carried out in tube cultures of KFBL cells. The cells were inoculated with serial 10-fold dilutions of a virus suspension, four tube cultures per dilution. The infectivity titer was calculated in $\log_{10}$ TCD_{50} per 0.1 ml by the method of Reed and Muench (10).

Plaque assays. For plaque assays, confluent monolayers of L-B or L-929 cells were cultivated in 60-mm plastic petri dishes at 37 C in 5% CO_2. Serial 10-fold dilutions of virus were allowed to adsorb to the cells for 45 min at 37 C. After virus adsorption, 4 ml of methylcellulose overlay, consisting of VM3 balanced salt solution, 0.2% glucose, 0.5% lactalbumine hydrolysate, 1% calf serum, and 0.75% methylcellulose (1), was added per plate. The plates were incubated for 5 days at 37 C in 5% CO_2. The overlay was then removed, and the cells were fixed with a 10% solution of Formalin and stained with undiluted Giemsa stain.

Inactivation with reduced DTT. DTT was obtained from Calbiochem Corp., Los Angeles, Calif. A fresh DTT solution in 0.01 M tris(hydroxymethyl)-aminomethane-hydrochloride buffer (pH 8.1) was prepared on the day of the experiment. The final DTT concentrations were 0.001 M or 0.002 M at pH 7.8. Drug-virus mixtures were incubated at 30 or 37 C. Samples were taken at different times of incubation and immediately placed in an ice bath to stop further inactivation. The infectivity of the samples was measured by end-point titrations (*see above*).

HA tests. The hemagglutinin of EAV for horse red blood cells (9) was titrated by the microtiter method. Serial twofold dilutions of a virus suspension in 0.05 ml of phosphate-buffered saline were made, and 0.05 ml of a 0.5% suspension of horse blood.cells was added to each dilution. The microtiter plates were kept at room temperature. The highest virus dilution showing complete hemagglutination (HA) was taken as the HA titer.

RESULTS

Kinetics of inactivation by DTT. Gainer et al. (6) showed that the rate of inactivation of pseudorabies virus by DTT was temperature dependent under mild alkaline conditions, being more rapid as the temperature was raised from 30 to 41 C.

The conditions of exposure of two different strains (419 and 647) of EAV to DTT were studied at two different concentrations of DTT (0.001 or 0.002 M) and at two different temperatures (30 and 37 C), at pH 7.8. At 37 C, both strains were inactivated within 60 to 75 min of exposure; the inactivation was rapid at both DTT concentrations used. At 30 C, the inactivation was slower than at 37 C so that inactivation curves could be obtained for both concentrations of DTT (Fig. 1 and 2). The inacti-

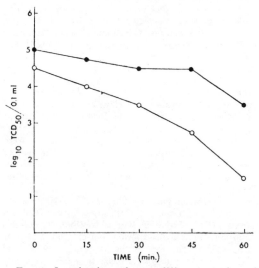

FIG. 1. *Inactivation of two different strains of equine abortion virus by 0.001 M DTT at 30 C and pH 7.8. Symbols:* ●, *vaccine strain RAC-H 419;* ○, *wild-type strain 647.*

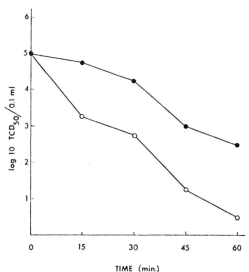

FIG. 2. *Inactivation of two different strains of equine abortion virus by 0.002 M DTT at 30 C and pH 7.8. Symbols:* ●, *vaccine strain RAC-H 419;* ○, *wild-type strain 647.*

vation was more rapid with 0.002 M DTT than with 0.001 M DTT. At both concentrations, the strains showed differences in sensitivity to DTT, the vaccine strain 419 being more resistant than the wild-type strain 647. Similar results were obtained with purified preparations of strains 419 and 647. These were used to ascertain that the inactivation by DTT was not influenced by nonviral constituents of the reaction mixture. Suspensions of untreated virus kept at 30 or 37 C and pH 7.8 had about the same titers throughout the test period.

Strain differences in the sensitivity to DTT. Since the vaccine strain 419 was more resistant to DTT than the wild-type strain 647, 13 additional wild-type strains were tested. The conditions of exposure were 0.002 M DTT for 30 min at 30 C and pH 7.8. The data in Table 1 show that, according to their sensitivity to DTT, the strains could be divided into three groups. Of all strains tested, strain 419 was the most resistant one. Strains SL-D and N-3 were placed in an intermediate group, whereas the remaining strains belong in the most sensitive group.

"L character" of EAV strains. Differences among EAV strains were described earlier by Borgen (1). The inability to produce plaques in

TABLE 1. *Grouping of equine abortion virus (EAV)*
strains by sensitivity to dithiothreitol (DTT)

EAV strain	Reduction in virus titer by DTT ($\log_{10}$ units TCD_{50})			L character[a]
	0-1	1-2	2-4	
RAC-H 419	0.75			L—
SL-D		1.25		L⁻
N-3		1.5		L⁻
RAC-H 17			3.0	L⁻
647			2.25	L⁺
488			2.25	L⁺
511			2.5	L⁺
463			2.5	L⁺
908			2.75	L⁺
1080			2.75	L⁺
510			3.0	L⁺
632			3.25	L⁺
825			3.25	L⁺
302			3.5	L⁺
800			3.5	L⁺

[a] Ability or inability to produce plaques in L-B cells (1).

L cells was considered as a marker for a few strains, including the vaccine strain RAC-H. We studied the ability of our strains to produce plaques in two different clones of L cells, L-B and L-929, respectively. In L-B cells the strains behaved as described by Borgen (1, 1a) whereas in L-929 cells all strains produced plaques with a plaque size of about 1 to 3 mm diameter. Strain 419 was characterized by two markers (Table 1), i.e., the inability to produce plaques in L-B cell monolayers, and relative resistance to DTT. Among the other strains, SL-D, N-3, and 17 were also unable to produce plaques in L-B cell monolayers but proved to be less resistant to DTT than strain 419.

Inactivation of EAV hemagglutinin by DTT. It was proposed that, in viruses sensitive to DTT, the protein coat of the virion became disrupted (6). The EAV hemagglutinin is supposedly located in the viral envelope. Therefore, we investigated whether the hemagglutinin is inactivated by DTT. Virus suspensions of strains 419 and 647, with a HA titer of 1:64 each, were incubated with 0.002 M DTT for 60 min at 30 C and pH 7.8. Samples of the virus suspensions were titrated for HA activity after different times of exposure to DTT. The results in Table 2 show that the hemagglutinins of both strains are inactivated at a similar rate. Untreated virus suspensions kept at 30 C and *p*H 7.8 have constant HA titers throughout the test period.

DISCUSSION

The high-passage derivative of the RAC-H strain was introduced as an attenuated, live vaccine against rhinopneumonitis and abortion in horses in West Germany (8). The importation of this vaccine strain to Sweden was made dependent on the fulfillment of certain requirements as, for instance, that for stable in vitro markers (5). In search for such markers, Borgen (1, 1a) described the inability of the vaccine RAC-H strain as well as of a few other strains (low-passage RAC-H, SL-D, N-3) to produce plaques in a clone of L cells, here called L-B. The majority of the strains tested were plaque producers in this cell line. In the present study, the findings of Borgen were confirmed as far as L-B cells were concerned. When another clone of L cells (L-929) was used, all strains did produce plaques. The difference between L-cell clones could not be explained.

In our search for markers, we found that the vaccine strain RAC-H is more resistant to inactivation by DTT than all other strains tested (Table 1). At present, the strain differences in sensitivity to DTT are difficult to explain. In studies on another herpesvirus, the pseudorabies virus, Gainer et al. (6) tried to explain the mechanism of inactivation by this drug. The main effect of DTT as determined by electron microscopy is disruption of the coat of the virion, probably due to cleavage of S-S linkages in cystine. Under similar conditions of exposure to DTT, the inactivation rate of the vaccine RAC-H strain is similar to that of the pseudorabies virus, whereas some of our other strains have proved to be much more sensitive to DTT than the pseudorabies virus.

The inactivation of hemagglutinin does support the notion that DTT interacts with and alters the envelope. However, the inactivation rates of the vaccine RAC-H strain and a wild-type strain are identical.

The vaccine RAC-H strain is characterized by two markers: a relative resistance to DTT (DTT marker) and the inability to produce plaques in L-B cells (L⁻ marker). The L⁻

marker is also found associated with the low-passage RAC-H strain, indicating that this marker is an intrinsic property of the RAC-H

TABLE 2. *Inactivation by dithiothreitol (DTT) of equine abortion virus (EAV) hemagglutinin*

EAV strain	HA titer[a] at time (min) of exposure to DTT				
	0	15	30	45	60
RAC-H 419	64	16	8	2	2
647	64	16	8	2	2

[a] Reciprocals of initial virus dilutions. HA, hemagglutinin.

strain (1). Since the vaccine RAC-H strain proves to be much more resistant to DTT than the low-passage RAC-H strain, it appears that this property may have been acquired during the course of numerous (419) passages in pig kidney cells. Thus, the L⁻ and DTT markers are not coupled properties, and the DTT marker does not necessarily indicate attenuation.

ACKNOWLEDGMENTS

The technical assistance of Maud Söderberg is gratefully acknowledged.

This investigation was supported by a grant from Svenska Travsällskapet.

LITERATURE CITED

1. Borgen, H. C. 1970. Differentiation of equine herpesvirus type 1 strains by a plaque marker. Arch. Gesamte Virusforsch. **32**:283–285.
1a. Borgen, H. C. 1972. Equine herpesvirus type 1; the L⁻ character in two of forty-three field isolates. Arch. Gesamte Virusforsch. **36**:391–393.
2. Carver, D. H., and D. S. Y. Seto. 1968. Viral inactivation by disulfide bond reducing agents. J. Virol. **2**: 1482–1484.
3. Cleland, W. W. 1964. Dithiothreitol, a new protective reagent for SH groups. Biochemistry **3**:480–482.
4. Diderholm, H., B. Stenkvist, J. Pontén, and T. Wesslén. 1965. Transformation of bovine cells in vitro after inoculation of simian virus 40 or its nucleic acid. Exp. Cell Res. **37**:452–459.
5. Dinter, Z. 1968. Live vaccine against equine abortion. Interim report to the Veterinary Board of Sweden. Dec. 1968 (in Swedish).
6. Gainer, J. H., J. Long, P. Hill, and W. I. Capps. 1971. Inactivation of the pseudorabies virus by dithiothreitol. Virology **45**:91–100.
7. Hare, J. D., and J. C. Chan. 1968. Role of hydrogen and disulfide bonds in polyoma capsid structure. Virology **34**:481–491.

7a. Klingeborn, B., and H. Pertoft. 1972. Equine abortion (herpes) virus: purification and concentration of enveloped and deenveloped virus and envelope material by density gradient centrifugation in colloidal silica. Virology **48**:618-623.

8. Mayr, A., J. Pette, K. Petzold, and K. Wagener. 1968. Untersuchungen zur Entwicklung eines Lebendimpfstoffes gegen die Rhinopneumonie (Stutenabort) der Pferde. Zentralbl. Veterinäermed. Reihe **15**:406-418.

9. McCollum, W. H., E. R. Doll, and J. T. Bryans. 1956. Agglutination of horse erythrocytes by tissue extracts from hamsters infected with equine abortion virus. Amer. J. Vet. Res. **17**:267-270.

10. Reed, L. J., and H. Muench. 1938. A simple method of estimating fifty percent endpoints. Amer. J. Hyg. **27**:493-497.

Thermal Resistance of Certain Oncogenic

Viruses Suspended in Milk and Milk Products

ROBERT SULLIVAN, JOHN T. TIERNEY, EDWARD P. LARKIN,

RALSTON B. READ, JR., AND JAMES T. PEELER

Thermal destruction rate curves were determined for adenovirus 12, reovirus 1, and herpes simplex virus in sterile milk, raw milk, raw chocolate milk, and raw ice cream mix. At 40 to 60 C, the curves were asymptotic to the base line. At 65 C, which is near the pasteurization standard, the curves approached a first-order reaction. Thermal resistance studies, by means of in vivo assays, of Moloney and Rauscher leukemia viruses and Moloney and Rous sarcoma viruses indicated that Rous sarcoma was the most resistant. A comparison of the 12D processes of Rous sarcoma virus, reovirus 1, adenovirus 12, and herpes simplex virus in ice cream mix (the most protective of the suspending menstrua studied) with the U.S. Public Health Service pasteurization standard indicated an adequate safety factor in current pasteurization practices.

Budding "C"-type viral particles have been observed in short-term phytohemagglutinin-stimulated lymphocytes recovered from the blood of normal and leukemic cattle (13). Similar viruses have been found in lymphocytes in cows' milk (12). Electron microscopic examination of feeder layers inoculated with buffy coats recovered from the blood of leukemic cattle and with long-term bovine lymphocyte suspension cultures revealed the presence of "C"-type budding viruses (4). Viruslike particles have also been found in milk, in biopsies, and in cell cultures derived from leukemic cows (7, 8, 10, 15, 20). These reports stimulated interest in viral heat resistance and thus in the adequacy of the pasteurization practices of the dairy industry.

Pasteurization times and temperatures recommended by the U.S. Public Health Service have been adopted by the states so that there is uniformity in the required minimal holding times and temperatures (21). The minimal standards are

(i) 62.8 C for 30 min or 71.7 C for 15 sec for milk, (ii) 65.6 C for 30 min or 74.4 C for 15 sec for milk products with added milk fat or sweeteners, and (iii) 68.3 C for 30 min or 79.4 C for 25 sec for ice cream mix.

Because the viruses demonstrated in milk and the lymphocytes could not be propagated in the laboratory, the assessment of the effectiveness of pasteurization was based on thermal inactivation studies of oncogenic animal viruses that could be assayed either in vivo or in vitro.

This report describes the thermal resistance of Rauscher and Moloney murine leukemia viruses, Moloney and Rous sarcoma viruses, adenovirus 12, herpes simplex virus, and reovirus 1 suspended in milk and milk products. Reovirus, although not a known tumor-producing virus, was studied because it has been isolated from human lymphoma (1, 17) and from feline leukemia patients (3, 16).

MATERIALS AND METHODS

Virus. Crude mouse spleen extracts of Rauscher leukemia virus, plasma concentrates of Moloney leukemia virus, partially purified extracts of Moloney sarcoma virus, and partially purified extracts of Rous sarcoma virus, Bryan strain, were obtained from various contractors within the Special Virus Cancer Program of the National Cancer Institute. In addition, adenovirus 12 NIAID, herpes simplex virus HF VR 260, and reovirus 1 Lang VR 230 were passaged in *Cercopithecus aethiops* primary kidney cell cultures.

In vitro assay. A modification of the plaque-forming unit assay previously developed was used in these studies (19). Viruses were assayed on primary cell cultures of *C. aethiops* monkey kidneys under an overlay medium. The medium contained 0.95% clarified Ionagar No. 2, Eagle's minimal essential medium with nonessential amino acids in Hanks balanced salt solution without phenol red, 2% fetal bovine serum, 0.19% $NaHCO_3$, 0.0015% neutral red dye, 0.51% $MgCl_2 \cdot 6H_2O$, and 1.0% sterile homogenized bovine milk. Bacterial and fungal contamination were controlled by the addition of 1,000 units of penicillin G, 1,000 mg of streptomycin sulfate, 50 μg of tetracycline hydrochloride, and 0.5 μg of amphotericin B per ml of the overlay medium. Plaques were counted and marked daily.

In vivo assay. The frozen ampoules containing the heat-treated leukemia viruses suspended in milk or ice cream mix were thawed in a water bath at 37 C. The contents of three ampoules were pooled and diluted with an equal volume of phosphate-buffered saline, and 0.1 ml was inoculated intraperitoneally into each of 20 Balb(c/cr) mice. Two additional 10-fold dilutions were made, and 20 mice were inoculated at each dilution. Unheated control samples, with and

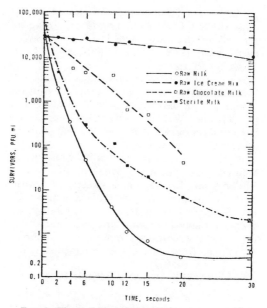
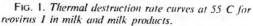

FIG. 1. *Thermal destruction rate curves at 55 C for reovirus 1 in milk and milk products.*

without virus, plus a standard virus control, were titrated with each sample tested. The test mice were less than 3 days old at the time of inoculation.

A toxic effect resulting in death of the mice within 48 hr was encountered when the samples were inoculated into the newborn mice. The minimal dilution that could be tolerated was $10^{-1.3}$. Therefore, all murine in vivo results were based on this dilution. The Rous sarcoma virus was diluted to 10^{-2} for similar reasons. The undiluted inoculum killed the embryos within 24 hr. Small numbers of viruses surviving the heat treatment could have been sufficiently diluted to prevent detection.

Mice inoculated with leukemia virus were palpated for splenomegaly or lymphadanopathy at weaning, and then at weekly intervals until they were sacrificed. All surviving animals were killed after 9 months.

With preparations containing Moloney sarcoma virus, mice were inoculated (0.1 ml) intramuscularly or subcutaneously in the left hind leg. The mice were examined for tumors at 7 days postinoculation and three times weekly thereafter. Surviving mice were killed after 4 months.

Serial dilutions of the Rous sarcoma virus preparations were inoculated onto the chorioallantoic membranes (CAM) of 9-day-old embryonated chicken eggs. After 10 days, the CAM were removed and the pocks were counted.

Histopathological examinations were performed on all mice that died or had abnormalities after inoculation with the terminal dilution samples.

Thermal inactivation. The virus was suspended in raw milk, sterile milk, raw chocolate milk, or raw ice cream mix, and was processed in a constant-temperature water bath or in a slug-flow heat exchanger (18). Tests at 40 to 60 C were made in the water bath for 5 to 30 min at 5-min intervals. High-temperature tests at 55 to 71.7 C at times ranging from 2 to 30 sec were processed in the heat exchanger.

Suspensions of adenovirus 12, herpes simplex virus, and reovirus 1 were diluted to obtain approximately 10^4 plaque-forming units per ml in the dairy product. The leukemia and sarcoma preparations were diluted 10^{-2} in the product to be examined. The resulting titers varied from $10^{2.3}$ to $10^{5.98}$ per ml depending on the lot used in the test. Ten replicates containing 1.2 ml of the suspension were tested at each temperature in the water bath method. Continuous agitation of the sample during the holding time was accomplished by means of a reciprocal shaker built into the bath. At the end of the heating times, the tubes were immediately cooled to 4 C, frozen, and stored at −65 C until tested. All samples for in vivo studies were shipped in dry ice to Microbiological Associates, Inc., Rockville, Md., for assay.

Corrections for the heating and residence time distribution effects in the heat exchanger have been previously reported (18). The time correction was 0.3 sec for low-viscosity fluids and 0.6 sec for the high-viscosity fluids. Such corrections, if calculated, would not

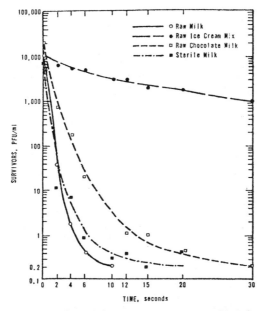

FIG. 2. *Thermal destruction rate curves at 55 C for herpes simplex virus in milk and milk products.*

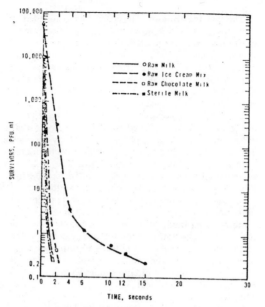

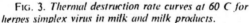

FIG. 3. *Thermal destruction rate curves at 60 C for herpes simplex virus in milk and milk products.*

affect the z values. Therefore, the calculations and corrections are not included in this report.

RESULTS

The destruction rate curves for reovirus 1 and herpes simplex virus at 55 C were asymptotic to the base line (Fig. 1 and 2). Similar results have been published for erythroblastosis virus, poliovirus 1, and rhinovirus HGP (2, 5, 9). The "tailing" effect was much less noticeable for herpes simplex virus at 60 C (Fig. 3). The destruction rate of herpes simplex virus appeared to approach a first-order reaction except when the virus was suspended in raw ice cream mix.

The asymptotic configuration was quite apparent with reovirus 1 at 60 C (Fig. 4). It was also apparent that the raw ice cream mix was the most protective medium of the dairy products studied.

At 65 C, the curves for adenovirus 12 and herpes simplex virus were first-order reactions (Fig. 5), and reovirus 1 appeared to be rapidly approaching this condition.

Calculation of the D values, the time required to reduce the viral concentration by 90%, was impossible, and the mechanism of thermal destruction is not known. However, it was feasible to employ the following polynomial mathematical

54

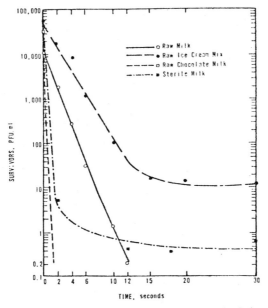

FIG. 4. *Thermal destruction rate curves at 60 C for reovirus 1 in milk and milk products.*

model to evaluate the consistency of plaque formation in repeated runs:

$$Y = \beta_0 + \beta_1 X + \beta_2 X^2 + \epsilon \qquad (1)$$

where Y equals $\log_{10}$ (plaque count/milliliter), β_0, β_1, and β_2 are true but unknown regression coefficients, X is time (minutes or seconds), and ϵ is experimental error. This model yielded adequate curve fits ($R^2 > 0.90$) in most experiments. A disadvantage of this model is that the regression coefficients cannot be easily related as a function of temperature.

An estimate of the relation between rate of inactivation and temperature was obtained by considering a conservative estimate of D. This D_I was based on the use of the inflection point estimate from equation 1. An example of this technique is presented in Fig. 6. The inflection point is $X_I = -b_1/2b_2$, where b_1 and b_2 are estimates of β_1 and β_2 in equation 1. Thus, a conservative estimate of D based on the X_I above is

$$D_I = \left| \frac{2}{b_1} \right| \qquad (2)$$

Values of z were computed in the usual manner with the use of D_I.

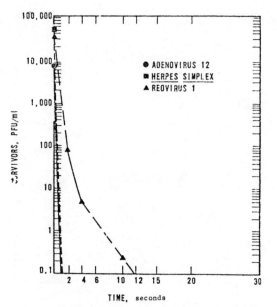

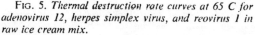

FIG. 5. *Thermal destruction rate curves at 65 C for adenovirus 12, herpes simplex virus, and reovirus 1 in raw ice cream mix.*

The D_1 value was determined for a sufficient number of runs at different temperatures so that z values could be calculated for all of the viruses in the in vitro study.

Results of the in vivo study of the resistance of Rauscher and Moloney leukemia viruses suspended in raw ice cream mix (the most protective of the dairy products) indicated that 50 C for 5 min or 55 C for 10 sec was sufficient to reduce the viral population so as to prevent leukemia, splenomegaly, or death in the inoculated mice. These results are comparable to data previously reported for Rauscher and Moloney leukemia viruses (14, 22).

The Moloney sarcoma virus was slightly more resistant than the leukemia viruses. Exposure for 15 min at 50 C or 20 sec at 55 C was sufficient to prevent the development of tumors in the inoculated mice.

Rous sarcoma virus appeared to be the most resistant of the viruses studied and survived at 55 C for 20 min and at 65 C for 2 sec. A half-life of 42 sec at 60 C has been previously reported (6).

The low initial titers of the viruses tested in vivo and the limitation in the amount of crude virus that could be added to the milk or milk product without adulterating or changing the thermal characteristics of the product presented difficulties when an attempt was made to analyze the results statistically. This problem was compounded by the necessity of diluting the viral inoculum because of adverse reactions in the newborn mouse and the embryonated chicken egg. Sufficient data, however, were available because of the relatively high initial titer of the Rous sarcoma virus preparations to calculate D values at four different temperatures. From these D values, the z value for Rous sarcoma could be plotted.

If a 12-log reduction, which is commonly used in industry to determine a food process, is utilized along with the calculated z values for Rous sarcoma virus, adenovirus 12, reovirus 1, and herpes simplex virus, a graphic comparison can be made with the U.S. Public Health Service pasteurization standard for ice cream mix (Fig. 7). It is apparent that the times and temperatures advocated by the U.S. Public Health Service for pasteurization of ice cream mix are sufficient to inactivate any of the oncogenic viruses tested. Theoretically, an ice cream mix suspension containing 12 logs of Rous sarcoma virus would be inactivated in 46 sec at 68.3 C (155 F) and in 1.4 sec at 79.4 C (175 F).

A lytic factor or nonspecific inhibitor of Rous

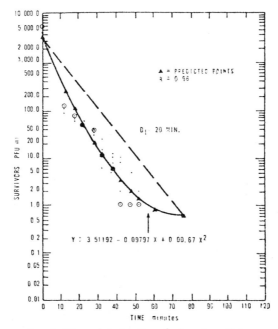

FIG. 6. *Thermal destruction of adenovirus 12 in raw milk at 52 C.*

sarcoma virus was present in three of the raw milk samples tested. The potency of this factor was such that a raw milk suspension containing 10^7 pock-forming units/ml was negative when inoculated onto the CAM of embryonated chicken eggs. Similar results were obtained with two other raw milk samples. Interestingly, the raw milk samples used in this study were all recovered from a bulk milk tank of a large milk-processing plant. A similar factor that reduced the titer of murine leukemia viruses has been reported (11).

DISCUSSION

The asymmetry of viral thermal destruction curves at low temperatures has been reported by other investigators. Whether survival is due to resistant members of the viral population or to the protective effect of the suspending menstruum is debatable. The destruction curves approached a first-order reaction as the temperatures studied neared the pasteurization temperatures. When the

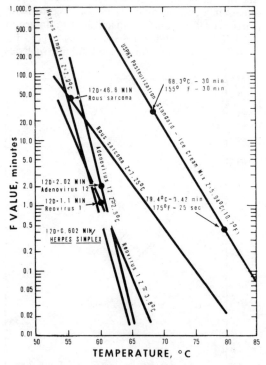

FIG. 7. *U.S. Public Health Service recommended pasteurization standard for ice cream mix compared to the thermal inactivation (12D) processes for Rous sarcoma, reovirus 1, adenovirus 12, and herpes simplex virus suspended in ice cream mix.*

58

z values were calculated for the viruses in the most protective medium, an adequate safety factor was present in the currently recommended pasteurization procedures. The calculated process, incorporating a 12D destruction factor, is greater than would be expected in milk or milk products. Unlike bacteria, viruses do not increase in numbers in milk. Therefore, the possibility of 12-log viral contamination is highly unlikely. Preliminary studies on the viral content of 57 raw milk samples indicated that viruses, if present at all, were present in small numbers. Viruses were found in two of the samples tested. Poliovirus 1 was recovered from one pooled sample and poliovirus 3 was recovered from the other sample (Sullivan et al., J. Dairy Sci. **52**:879, 1966).

Whether similar results would be obtained with the reported bovine viruses can only be determined with the development of an assay system that will make possible a similar study to determine the thermal inactivation properties of these agents.

The presence of an interfering factor for Rous sarcoma virus in three samples of raw milk raises questions as to the possible presence of antibodies to a bovine oncogenic virus or to an avian tumor virus in cows' milk. An attempt should be made to determine a possible relationship of this factor to a subclinical infection of bovine leukemia.

ACKNOWLEDGMENTS

This research was supported by research project NCI-VCL-(65)-30 within the special virus cancer program, National Cancer Institute.

The in vivo assays were performed by Gerald Spahn, Microbiological Associates, Inc., under contract PH 43-67-697 from the special virus cancer program, National Cancer Institute.

LITERATURE CITED

1. Anonymous. 1968. Reappraisal of Burkett's lymphoma. Brit Med. J. **1**:332.
2. Bonar, R. A., D. Beard, G. S. Beaudreau, G. D. Sharp, and J. W. Beard. 1957. Virus of avian erythroblastosis. IV. pH and thermal stability. J. Nat. Cancer Inst. **18**:831-842.
3. Burger, C. L., and F. Noronha. 1970. Feline leukemia virus: purification from tissue culture fluids. J. Nat. Cancer Inst. **45**:499-503.
4. Cornefert-Jensen, F., W. C. D. Hare, and N. D. Stock. 1969. Studies on bovine lymphosarcoma: formation of syncytia and detection of virus particles in mixed-cell cultures. Int. J. Cancer **4**:507-519.
5. Dimmock, N. J. 1967. Differences between the thermal inactivation of picornaviruses at "high" and "low" temperatures. Virology **31**:338-353.
6. Dougherty, R. M. 1961. Heat inactivation of Rous sarcoma virus. Virology **14**:371-372.
7. Dutcher, R. M. 1965. Bovine leukemia. Growth **29**:1-5.

8. Dutcher, R. M., E. P. Larkin, and R. R. Marshak. 1964. Virus-like particles from cow's milk from a herd with a high incidence of lymphosarcoma. J. Nat. Cancer Inst. 33:1055–1064.

9. Eckert, E. A., I. Green, D. G. Sharp, D. Beard, and J. W. Beard. 1955. Virus of erythromyeloblastic leukosis. VII. Thermal stability of virus infectivity; the virus particle; and the enzyme diphosphorylating adenosinetriphosphate. J. Nat. Cancer Inst. 16:153–161.

10. Jensen, E. M., and G. Shidlowsky. 1964. Submicroscopic particles in normal bovine and human milks: a preliminary morphological report. J. Nat. Cancer Inst. 33:1029–1053.

11. Larkin, E. P., and R. M. Dutcher. 1970. Recovery of Rauscher leukemia virus from large volumes of seeded cow's milk and from infected murine spleens. Appl. Microbiol. 20:64–68.

12. Malmquist, W. A., M. J. Van Der Maaten, and A. D. Boothe. 1969. Isolation, immunodiffusion, immunfluorescence, and electron microscopy of a syncytial virus of lymphosarcomatous and apparently normal cattle. Cancer Res. 29:188–200.

13. Miller, J. M., L. D. Miller, C. Olson, and K. G. Gillette. 1969. Virus-like particles in phytohemagglutinin-stimulated cultures with reference to lymphosarcoma. J. Nat. Cancer Inst. 43:1297–1305.

14. Moloney, J. B. 1962. The murine leukemias. Fed. Proc. 21:19–31.

15. Nazerian, K., R. M. Dutcher, E. P. Larkin, J. J. Tumilowicz, and C. P. Eusebio. 1968. Elecron microscopy of virus-like particles found in bovine leukemia. Amer. J. Vet. Res. 29:387–395.

16. Rickard, C. G., J. E. Post, F. Noronha, and L. Barr. 1969. A transmissible, virus-induced leukemia of the cat. J. Nat. Cancer Inst. 42:987–1014.

17. Stanley, N. F. 1967. Reoviruses. Brit. Med. Bull. 23:150–155.

18. Stroup, W. H., R. W. Dickerson, Jr., and R. B. Read, Jr. 1969. Two-phase slug flow heat exchanger for microbial thermal inactivation research. Appl. Microbiol. 18:889–892.

19. Sullivan, R., and R. B. Read, Jr. 1968. Method for the recovery of viruses from milk and milk products. J. Dairy Sci. 51:1748–1751.

20. Tumilowicz, J. J., and S. Shirahama. 1969. Aberrant characteristics of virus-like particles in bovine mammary cell cultures. Amer. J. Vet. Res. 30:51–59.

21. U.S. Department of Health, Education, and Welfare. 1965. Grade "A" Pasteurized Milk Ordinance. U.S. Public Health Serv. Publ. 229.

22. Zeigel, R. F., and F. J. Rauscher. 1964. Electron microscopic and bioassay studies on a murine leukemia virus (Rauscher). I. Effects of physiochemical treatments on the morphology and biological activity of the virus. J. Nat. Cancer Inst. 32:1277–1307.

INHIBITION OF HERPES VIRUS ADSORPTION BY TWO FRACTIONS OBTAINED FROM COMMERCIAL PROTAMINE SULFATE

SHIGERU YAMAMOTO, HIDEFUMI KABUTA
AND YOH NAKAGAWA

The commercial protamine sulfate could be separated into two fractions by Sephadex G-50 column which inhibited plaque formation by herpes simplex virus when cell monolayers were treated with them before adding the virus. One of them (Fr. I) contains high molecular weight proteins and the other (Fr. II) contains only protamine molecules. The former is more effective than the latter. The inhibitory effect disappears after incubation of the fractions with a large amount of cells. Both fractions do not directly reduce virus infectivity. Furthermore, they do not inhibit virus replication after virus adsorption. The virus particles remaining unadsorbed to cells pretreated with the fractions could be detected only when virus diluted in Earle's saline containing skim milk and lactalbumin hydrolysate was used for inoculation. These findings gave a clear evidence that protamine (Fr. II) and also high molecular weight proteins in Fr. I adsorb to cell surface or receptor and in consequence inhibit virus attachment to the cell surface resulting in the reduction of plaque formation.

The basic proteins and the synthetic basic polymers affect the interaction of virus or viral RNA with cells although they are different in effect among a variety of viruses. In some cases they interfere with the virus-cell interaction[3][4][13], but in others enhance it[1][9][11][12][14]. Recently, the contrasting effects were found even between two variants of encephalomyocarditis virus[5]. It was revealed in the previous report that the plaque formation by herpes simplex virus was also reduced if the cell monolayers were exposed to protamine sulfate before inoculation with the virus[17]. It has been found that the commercial protamine sulfate can be separated into two protein fractions by gel filtration. This paper deals with the comparison of effects of the two fractions on virus-cell interaction, and the evidence obtained here demonstrates that both fractions bind to the cell surface and inhibit the adsorption of virus particles to cell resulting in the reduction of plaque formation.

MATERIALS AND METHODS

Cells. G-7 cells, a clone isolated from GMK cells (established African grivet monkey kidney cells), were grown in 2-oz bottles with approximately one million cells using a mixture consisting of 7 parts of Hank's saline containing 0.5 % lactalbumin hydrolysate and 3 parts of Eagle's medium, supplemented with 10 % heated (56 °C, 30 minutes) bovine serum.

Virus. The M strain of herpes simplex virus had been transfered ten times in GMK cell cultures following its isolation from a case with Herpes labialis. Characteristics of this strain have been described previously [8] [16].

Solution. Phosphate-buffered saline, pH 7.2 (PBS), and that deprived of $MgCl_2$ and $CaCl_2$ (PBS(−)) were prepared according to Dulbecco and Vogt[6]. Earle's saline supplemented with 0.5 % skim milk and 0.125 % lactalbumin hydrolysate (MLE) was used in some experiments.

Protamine. Protamine sulfate (salmine) was obtained from Nutritional Biochemicals Corp.

62

Fractionation of protamine sulfate by Sephadex. Protamine sulfate was dissolved in PBS(−) at a concentration of 50 mg/ml and yielded a turbid solution which was centrifuged at 10,000 r. p. m for ten minutes at 25 to 28 °C, and filtered through a 0.22 μ Millipore filter. Two to four ml of the filtrate were applied on Sephadex G-50 column, 2 × 20 cm, and eluted with PBS (−).

Protein estimation. The protein content in each fraction was measured by the method of Lowry et al.[10] using bovine albumin as a standerd.

Treatment of cell monolayers with the fractions. The two-day old monolayer cultures were washed twice with five ml PBS. The washed monolayers were exposed to five ml of the fraction appropriately diluted with PBS for one hour at 37 °C. Control cultrures were exposed to PBS under the same conditions. The cultures were then washed twice with PBS and followed by standing in five ml PBS for 30 minutes at room temperature to remove completely the substances in the fraction from culture bottles. After the fluid was drained off, the monolayers were inoculated with two tenth ml of virus suspension in PBS containing 50 to 100 PFU (plaque forming units). Four to five bottle cultures were used for one titration. The virus was allowed to adsorb for two hours at 37 °C and overlaid according to the method as described previously[16].

RESULTS

Fractionation of protamine sulfate by Sephadex G-50 and the effect on plaque formation. Two ml of protamine sulfate solution were applied to Sephadex G-50 column. Fractions of two ml were collected and diluted with

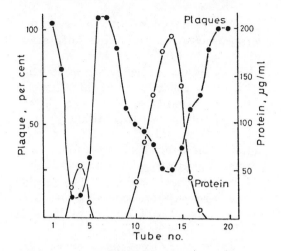

Fig. 1 Fractionation of protamine sulfate
by Sephadex G-50.

Two ml of protamine solution were applied on the column, 2×20 cm, and eluted
with PBS (−). The first 15 ml were discard-
ed. Every fraction (2 ml) was diluted 25 times
with PBS and used for treatment of cell
monolayers. Aliquots from diluted fractions
were assayed for protein content.

48 ml PBS and the effect on plaque
formation was tested. At the same
time, aliquots from the diluted fractions
were assayed for protein content. As
illustrated in Fig. 1, two peaks of
protein were obtained and the first one
was more effective on the reduction in
the number of plaques formed by M
strain than the second peak, although
it contained smaller amount of protein
than the other. In addition, no alteration of plaque characteristics was
observed with these peaks. The first
peak appeared also in excluded fraction
when it was rechromatographed through
the column of Sephadex G-100.

The tubes 3 to 5 and 12 to 14 were
pooled and referred to as Fr. I and Fr.
II, respectively, for the following experiments. As the eluants appearing after
the tube 15 were contaminated with
excess of SO_4^{--} ions derived from the
original solution of protamine sulfate,

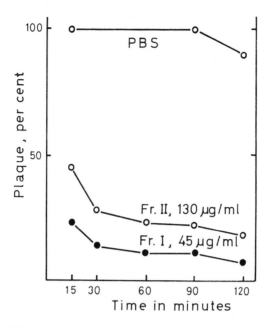

Fig. 2 Effect of the exposure time on plaquing efficiency.
Cell monolayers were incubated with Fr.
I or Fr. II for the indicated period before
addition of virus.

they were not used for experiments.

*Effect of the exposure time on
plaque reduction.* The washed monolayers were exposed to 45 and 130 μg/ml
of Fr. I and Fr. II, respectively, and
PBS at 37 °C. At the given time, the
monolayers were washed and tested on
plaque formation. Fig. 2 indicated that
maximum reduction was achieved at 30
minutes in both cases. Incubation over
90 minutes reduced the number of
plaques in the control monolayers which
were exposed to PBS. Therefore, the
incubation for 60 minutes seems to be
adequate for estimating the reduction
of plaques by Fr. I or Fr. II.

Reduction of plaques by various concentrations of Fr. I and Fr. II.

The relationship between the concentration of Fr. I or Fr. II with which the cell monolayers were treated and the number of plaques formed were illustrated in Fig. 3. Below the concentration of 6 μg/ml, the reduction of the number of plaques was not so different between Fr. I and Fr. II, whereas, over this concentration, Fr. I markedly reduced the number of plaques formed in comparison with Fr. II. The effetiveness of Fr. I was not enhanced by increasing the concentration at higher than 50 μg/ml. Fr. I and Fr. II were not toxic to cells at the concentration lower than 200 μg/ml.

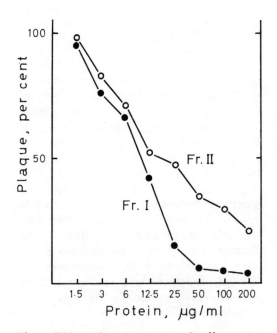

Fig. 3 Effect of pretreatment of cell monolayers with different concentrations of Fr. I and Fr. II on plaquing efficiency.

Effect of Fr. I and Fr. II on virus infectivity. The virus suspension which contained approximately 5×10^7 PFU/ml was mixed with an equal volume of PBS, 2 mg/ml of Fr. I and Fr. II. After incubation for one hour at 37°C with shaking, the mixture was diluted 100,000 times and inoculated on to the cell monolayers for plaque assay. The trace amount of Fr. I and Fr. II remaining in diluted mixtures should be too low in the concentration to affect the plaque formation. The PFUs of the diluted mixtures treated with Fr. I , Fr. II and PBS were 198.5, 176.5 and 191.5 per ml, respectively. The values are not significantly different indicating that the virus particle is not inactivated by either Fr. I or Fr. II.

Effect of Fr. I and Fr. II on virus replication. Monolayer cultures were washed twice with PBS and inoculated with 0.2 ml virus suspension. The inoculum contained 3 PFU per cell, which were allowed to adsorb for two hours at 37°C. The cell monolayers were then washed five times with PBS and incubated at 37°C in four ml of Eagle's medium or of that containing 25 μg/ml of Fr. I or Fr. II. At each time interval indicated in Fig. 4, the cultures were frozen and thawed and followed by sonication for two minutes at 20 kc/sec. Fig. 4 shows that both fractions do not affect or slightly enhance virus replication after virus adsorption. Maximum yield of virus was observed 21 hours after adsorption in every case, and at this time more virus was found in cultures with Fr. I and Fr. II than in control (1200, 1300 and 850 PFU per cell, respectively).

Adsorption of Fr. I and Fr. II with cells. An experiment was designed to see if there was a possibility that the

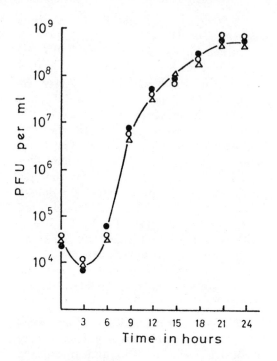

Fig. 4 Virus replication in the presence of Fr. I and Fr. II.

Cells were inoculated with virus at a multiplicity of 3 PFU per cell. After adsorption for two hours, the cultures were washed five times and incubated at 37°C in four ml medium. At the time intervals indicated, the virus was harvested and assayed. The media were Eagle's medium (△), Eagle's medium containing 25μg/ml of Fr. I (•) and Eagle's medium containing 25 μg/ml of Fr. II (○).

substances in Fr. I and Fr. II may bind to cell surface and result in the inhibition of virus attachment to the cell. The cells were dispersed by trypsin and washed twice with a large amount of PBS. The cells were suspended to give a suspension containing 5×10^7 cells in 25 ml of PBS, Fr. I and Fr. II (15 μg/ml), and incubated at 37°C for one hour with intermittent shaking. After incubation, the suspension was centrifuged to remove cells and the supernatant fluid was added to cell monolayers in order to see the effect on plaque formation. Further adsorption, when necessary, was carried out by the same procedure as above. The results are shown in Table 1. It is clear that the plaque reducing effect of Fr. I was completely diminished by preincubation with cells, while five cycles of adsorption were required to reverse the inhibitory effect of Fr. II. The result may be attributed to the difference in molecular size of substances contained in Fr. II. As the behavior in Sephadex column showed that the substances in Fr. II was lower molecular size than those in Fr. I, the concentration in Fr. II may be higher on a molar basis. This may accordingly result in the requirement of larger amount of cells for adsorbing the substances in Fr. II.

Fate of unadsorbed virus. An attempt was made to study the fate of the virus particles. The inoculum which was adsorbed for two hours on cell monolayers pretreated with PBS, Fr. I or Fr. II (25 μg/ml) was removed and transferred to fresh cultures for estimation of unadsorbed virus. The virus for inoculation was diluted in PBS in one experiment, and in MLE in the other one. As shown in Table 2, when the virus in PBS was used, the amount of virus remaining in the inoculum applied to monolayers pretreated with Fr. I was significantly less than the control and that in the case of Fr. II was roughly comparable to it.

When the virus diluted in MLE was inoculated on to the cells pretreated with Fr. I and Fr. II, the plaquing efficiencies were 26 and 86%, respectively (Table 2, Expt. 2). These values are higher than those obtained in the experiment which carried out with the

69

TABLE 1

Effect of adsorption of Fr. I and Fr. II with cells on plaquing efficiency

	Before adsorption		After adsorption	
	av. no. of plaques	plaquing efficiency	av. no. of plaques	plaquing efficiency
Expt. 1			adsorbed 1× with cells	
Fr. I, 15 µg/ml	39.3	33	118.4	107
Fr. II, 15 µg/ml	51.4	44	55.0	50
PBS	118.2	100	110.0	100
Expt. 2			adsorbed 5× with cells	
Fr. II, 15 µg/ml	51.3	55	77.0	86
PBS	93.0	100	89.3	100

Adsorption was carried out by incubating the suspension of 5×10^7 cells in 25 ml of Fr. I, Fr. II and PBS at 37°C for one hour.

TABLE 2
Inhibitory effect of pretreatment of cell monolayers on virus adsorption

Pretreatment of cultures with	Inoculation with virus in	Adsorbed virus		Unadsorbed virus		Recovery %
		total PFU	Plaquing efficiency	total PFU	% of control	
Expt. 1						
Fr. I, 25 µg/ml	PBS	59	14	61	80	24
Fr. II, 25 µg/ml	"	209	50	84	111	60
PBS	"	415	100	76	100	100
Expt. 2						
Fr. I, 25 µg/ml	MLE	189	26	201	216	48
Fr. II, 25 µg/ml	"	615	86	168	181	97
PBS	"	714	100	93	100	100

After adsorption of virus to treated and untreated cell monolayers, the inoculum was removed and transferred to fresh cultures to estimate unadsorbed virus. For estimation of adsorbed virus, the cultures were overlaid immediately after removal of the inoculum.

71

virus diluted in PBS (Table 2, Expt. 1). The reason is not clear but it seems that MLE can partially reduce the inhibitory effect probably by masking the substances contained in the fractions which previously adsorbed to the cell surface or by releasing them from the cell surface by competition with their binding site. In fact, MLE reacts with Fr. I and Fr. II and the precipitate is produced. Repeated experiments on Fr. II (25 μg/ml) using the virus diluted in MLE showed the plaquing efficiencies to be 75 to 88 %. Therefore, 86 % plaquing efficiency (i. e, 14 % reduction) seems to be significant although the difference from control is small.

Furthermore, more numbers of PFU were detected in the inocula which were applied to monolayers pretreated with Fr. I and Fr. II in comparison with the control. These results clearly demonstrate that substances in Fr. I and Fr. II inhibit adsorption of virus particles to cell surface resulting in the reduction of plaques. On the other hand, the discrepancy of the results with the unadsorbed virus obtained between experiments which were carried out with the virus in PBS and with that in MLE seems worthy of consideration.

One possibility is that the virus particles remaining unadsorbed in the inoculum may be inactivated more rapidly in PBS than in MLE under the condition of the temperature of 37°C during adsorption period.

There exists another possibility that some component might be released from pretreated cells which would inactivate unadsorbed virus particles in PBS but not those in MLE. To test this possibility, the following experiments were undertaken. Two-tenth ml PBS were added to cell cultures pretreated with

Fr. I , Fr. II and PBS. After incubation for two hours at 37°C, the 'conditioned' fluid was collected and diluted two-fold stepwise with PBS after centrifugation. In one experiment, 0.3 ml dilutions of the conditioned fluid were mixed with 0.3 ml PBS and incubated at 37°C for 30 minutes and then 0.6 ml of virus suspension appropyriatel diluted in PBS were added. After further incubation for 30 minutes at 37 or 25°C, infectivities were determined. The other experiment was carried out by the same procedures except that 0.3 ml dilutions of the conditioned fluid were mixed with 0.3 ml MLE instead of PBS. As shown in Table 3, the conditioned fluid from PBS - treated cells is as effective as MLE in protecting virus and the protection decreases by dilution unless MLE is added in the fluid. However, the conditioned fluid from Fr. I - or Fr. II - treated cells inhibit weakly but significantly virus infectivity. It is evident that this inhibitory effect is not due to the interference with virus adsorption to cell surface at the time of plaque assay since the pretreatment of cell monolayers with the conditioned fluid from Fr. I - or Fr. II -treated cells does not affect the plaque formation as shown in Table 4. On the other hand, addition of MLE reverse the inhibition by the conditioned fluid from Fr. II but cannot reverse the inhibition by the conditioned fluid from Fr. I . These results leads to a speculation that the cells treated with Fr. I or Fr. II release some factor into fluid which inhibit virus infectivity. Some component in MLE may probably combine with such an inhibitor released from Fr. II - treated cells making the inhibitor inactive, whereas, it does not affect the inhibitor from Fr. I -treated

TABLE 3

Effect of "conditioned" fluid from pretreated cell monolayers
on virus infectivity

Final dilution of conditioned fluid	Conditioned fluid from cells pretreated with					
	Fr. I		Fr. II		PBS	
	Preincubation with					
	PBS	MLE	PBS	MLE	PBS	MLE
Expt. 1						
1 : 4	70	71	69	90	86	94
1 : 8	62	74	59	91	78	92
1 : 16	45	71	48	99	66	94
1 : 32	40	70	47	101	66	100
1 : 64	17	81	26	101	56	95
Expt. 2						
1 : 4	73	72			100	94
1 : 8	102	97			102	100
1 : 16	96	98			101	100
1 : 32	84	100			82	99

Conditioned Fluid was obtained by incubating cell monolayers pretreated with Fr. I,
Fr. II (25 μg/ml) and PBS in 0.2 ml PBS per culture bottle.

Three-tenth ml of diluted conditioned fluid was mixed with an equal voloume of PBS
or MLE, and incubated at 37°C for 30 minutes (Preincubation). Further incubation at
37°C (Expt. 1) or 25°C (Expt. 2) was done after adding 0.6 ml virus diluted in PBS.

The numbers represent per cent infectivities of control. Infectivity of control, which
contained PBS instead of the conditioned fluid and was kept in ice water, was 75.2 PFU/0.2 ml.

74

TABLE 4

*Effect of pretreatment of cell monolayers with "conditioned" fluid
on plaquing effeciency*

Pretreatment of cell monolayers with conditioned fluid from cells treated with	Av. no. of Plaques	Plaquing efficiency
Fr. I	88.0	102
Fr. II	93.0	107
PBS	87.0	100
Control[a]	86.5	100

Conditioned fluid was obtained as described in Table 3.
Cell monolayers were treated with 1 : 2 dilution of the
conditioned fluid before adding the virus.
a) Cell monolayers pretreated with PBS.

cells. Such an event accounts for the finding in preceding experiment (Table 2, Expt. 2) that, when virus in MLE was used for inoculation, practically the same recovery (total amount of adsorbed and unasorbed virus particles) was obtained in cell monolayers pretreated with Fr. II as in control monolayers, but only lower recovery in cell monolayers pretreated with Fr. I .

Effect of Fr. I and Fr II on virus clones. An experiment was carried out to confirm whether the reduction of plaques in pretreated monolayers was caused by some variants possibly contaminated in virus inoculum. Virus clones were isolated from the single plaques formed by adsorbed and unadsorbed virus to cell monolayers which were treated with PBS, Fr. I and Fr. II (Table 2, Expt. 2). Each clone was propagated passing once in cells, and tested on the plaque forming ability in treated or untreated cell monolayers. As shown in Table 5, the reduction of plaques formed in pretreated monolayers

TABLE 5

Effect of Fr. I and Fr. I on plaquing efficiency of virus clones derived from different origins

Clones derived from	no. of clones	Plaquing efficiency in cell monolayers pretreated with 20 µg/ml of	
		Fr. I	Fr. II
virus adsorbed to cells pretreated with Fr. I	4	19-28 (23)	57-73 (62)
" Fr. II	5	16-26 (20)	48-84 (66)
" PBS	5	20-27 (24)	47-75 (68)
virus unadsorbed to cells pretreated with Fr. I	8	12-28 (19)	40-73 (55)
" Fr. II	8	17-25 (20)	43-81 (61)
" PBS	7	16-28 (19)	44-81 (64)

Numbers in parenthesis represent the average values of plaquing efficiencies.

were roughly comparable in clones regardless of their origins. It is, therefore, unlikely that the virus stock consisted of the mixed populations which contained variants with and without ability to attach to the pretreated cells.

Effect of heating on Fr. I and Fr. II. Fr. I and Fr. II (1 mg/ml) in PBS (−) were heated at different temperatures and exposed to cell monolayers after being diluted 40 times with PBS (25 μg/ml in final concentration). The plaque reducing capacity of Fr. I and II was maintained after heating at 56°C for 30 minutes. As shown in Fig. 5, Fr. II was very stable for heating at 100°C. In contrast, Fr. I rapidly but partially lost the plaque reducing capacity at 100°C, and maintained it thereafter at a constant level.

Digestion of Fr. I and Fr. II by trypsin. Two ml of PBS (−), Fr. I and Fr. II in PBS (−) were mixed with equal volume of 0.3 % trypsin (DIFCO, 1 : 250) in 0.02 M Tris (tris (hydroxymethyl) aminomethane) buffer, pH 8.0, and incubated at 37°C. After digestion for two hours, the mixture was heated in boiling water for five minutes to inactivate the enzyme. The mixtures were diluted 7 times with PBS and used for estimation of plaque reduction.

Table 6 shows that the numbers of plaques formed in cell monolayers treated with trypsin-digested Fr. I and Fr. II were as same as control. As Fr. I was partially heat labile (Fig. 5), another experiment in which the enzyme was inactivated by adding the bovine serum into reaction mixture after incubation was attempted and the same result was obtained. This clearly pointed out that the plaque reducing capacity was associated to the protein or protein moiety in substances contained in Fr. I and Fr. II.

TABLE 6

Effect of trypsin-digested Fr. I and Fr. II on plaquing efficiency

Pretreatment of cultures with	Av. no. of plaques	Plaquing efficiency
PBS (−)	103.6	100
" treated with trypsin	115.0	100
Fr. I, 25 μg/ml	15.6	15
" treated with trypsin	124.6	108
Fr. II, 150 μg/ml	25.6	25
" treated with trypsin	117.2	102

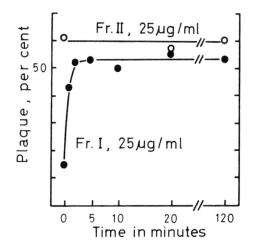

Fig. 5 Effect of heating on plaque reducing
capacity of Fr. I and Fr. II.

Fr. I and Fr. II containing 1 mg protein
per ml in PBS (−) were heated in boiling
water for indicated period. The cell monolayers were treated with heated sample after
diluted 40 times with PBS.

*Amino acid composition of Fr. I
and Fr. II.* The qualitative amino
acid analysis was carried out by two-
dimensional paper chromatography on
acid hydrolysates of Fr. I and Fr. II.
Fr. I and Fr. II were desalted by
eluting with distilled water through
Sephadex G-10 column and hydrolyzed
by 6 N HCl at 110 °C for 16 hours in
sealed ampules filled with nitrogen gas.
The hydrolysates were condensed under
reduced pressure and served for chromatography. Phenol-water containing
1% ammonia (4 : 1) and n-butanol-acetic
acid-water (4 : 1 : 2) were used as
developing solvents. Fourteen spots
corresponding to amino acids and two
unidentified spots were clearly separated on the chromatogram of hydrolysate
of Fr. I. On the other hand, only
seven spots were recognized in the
hydrolysate of Fr. II. Those were iso-

leucine-phenylalanine, valine-methioni-
ne, alanine, glycine, serine, proline and
arginine, among which the spot of
arginine was especially large and intense
in color. The relatively small amount
of arginine was detected in Fr. I by
visual comparison of spots on the chromatogram. This was also confirmed by
Sakaguchi reaction[7] carried out on the
paper. The result obtained on Fr. II
was in accord with the amino acid
analysis of salmine reported by Ando
et al[2]. It is, thus, confirmed that
Fr. II contains only protamine molecules.
The behavior in Sephadex column and
the amino acid analysis clearly demonstrates that Fr. I does not contain the
aggregates of protamine molecules but
is composed of different protein(s) with
higher molecular weight.

DISCUSSION

The commercial protamine sulfate
could be separated into two fractions
by Sephadex G-50 column which inhibited the virus-cell interation, one of
which (Fr. I) contains high molecular
weight protein(s) and the other (Fr. II)
contains only protamine molecules.
Both fractions inhibit the plaque formation by herpes simplex virus in cell
monolayers if the cells are treated with
them before inoculation with the virus,
although Fr. I inhibits much more
efficiently than does Fr. II. As the
plaque reducing capacity of Fr. I is
partially diminished by heating, it
may be reasonable to consider that it
contains several kinds of proteins.
Wallis and Melnick[15] found that
protamine sulfate increased the number
and the size of plaques formed by
herpes simplex virus when it was
introduced in agar overlay medium.

80

Our previous study showed that it slightly increased the size of plaques but did not affect the number of plaques when it was introduced in agar[16]. In the present experiment, it was confirmed that Fr. I and Fr. II did not affect or slightly enhanced virus replication when either of the fractions was added in the medium after virus adsorption (Fig. 4) and that they did not directly affect virus infectivity.

On the other hand, if the cells are treated with the fractions before adding the virus, the number of plaques is reduced (Fig. 1). These findings lead to the assumption that the fractions neither inactivate the intra- and extracellular virus nor inhibit virus replication but they bind to the cell surface and in consequence prevent virus attachment to or inactivate virus on the cell surface. Binding of the substances to cells could be clearly demonstrated by removal of plaque reducing capacity of Fr. I and II by preincubation with cells (Table 1). The fact that the plaque reduction is due to the failure of virus attachment to pretreated cells became evident from experiments in which the number of PFU remaining in inoculum was determined after adsorption period (Table 2). This strongly supports the hypothesis proposed by Colter et al.[3] and by Craighead and Layne[5] that polycations block the receptor site by binding to the cell surface.

Craighead and Layne[5] failed to recover the unadsorbed virus from the inoculum which was applied to polycation-treated monolayers. In our experiment, such unadsorbed virus could be detected only when the virus diluted in MLE was used for inoculation but could not detected when the virus diluted in

PBS was used. The data obtained here indicate that some factor will be released from cells pretreated with Fr. II which inactivate virus but could not inactivate it in MLE (Table 3). Although such a factor has not yet been characterized, it seems probably that it is the complex of protamine molecule and cell receptor, which, if it is once released into fluid will be capable of binding to virus particle and will result in inactivation of virus. Such a complex will be also capable of binding to some substances, probably protein or peptide, which are contained in skim milk or lactalbumin hydrolysate, and in consequence will diminish its capacity of binding to virus particle. In the case of Fr. I, a similar complex will be released but not affected by MLE.

Protamine enhances adsorption of P[32]-labelled fowl plague virus to cells[1] and DEAE dextran enhances infectivity of poliovirus and its infectious RNA[12]. The infectivity of rabies virus is remarkably enhanced by protamine or DEAE dextran[9] and that of respiratory syncytial virus is also enhanced by DEAE dextran and by low concentration of protamine[11]. On the other hand, protamine reduces infectivity of Semliki Forest virus but increases RNA infectivity[4]. In addition, infection of mengo encephalomyelitis virus is inhibited by protamine[3]. Our preliminary experiments showed that protamine enhanced markedly the plaque formation by measles virus and to a lesser extent by poliovirus, but reduced that by Sindbis virus. Such the contrasting effects of polycations among various viruses are probably due to the differences of surface structure of virus particles. Many authors have attributed the effects of polycations on virus infectivity to ionic charge. The experiment on a variant of encephalomyocarditis virus by Craighead and Layne supports this hypothesis[5]. They observed that plaque formation by r^+ variant was inhibited by basic polyamino acid to a greater degree at low than high pH values. However, our repeated experiments by using Fr. I and II and herpes simplex virus carried out by strictly the same manner did not give the results comparable to that obtained by them. It seems, therefore, unlikely to consider that the ionic charge is the sole factor in the effect of polycations on virus adsorption or infectivity.

Although no evidence was obtained that Fr. I and II affect the virus-cell interaction by the different mechanism, the data obtained here demonstrate that both fraction inhibit virus adsorption by binding to the cell surface. However, the biochemical mechanism by which the virus-cell interaction is inhibited still remains to be elucidated.

LITERATURE CITED

1) ALLISON, A. C. and VALENTINE, R. C. : Virus particle adsorption Ⅲ. Adsorption of viruses by cell monolayers and effects of some variables on adsorption. Biochim. Biophys. Acta., **40**, 400-410, 1960.

2) ANDO, T., ISHII, S. and SATO, M. : Studies on protamines Ⅵ. Amino acid composition of clupeine and salmine. J. Biochem., **46**, 933-940, 1959.

3) COLTER, J. S., DAVIES, M. A. and CAMPBELL, J. B. : Studies of three variants of mengo encephalomyelitis virus. Ⅰ. Inhibition of interaction with L cells by an agar inhibitor and by protamine. Virology, **24**, 578-585, 1964.

4) CONNOLLY, J. H. : Effect of histones and protamine on the infectivity of Semliki Forest virus and its ribonucleic acid. Nature, **212**, 858, 1966.

83

5) CRAIGHEAD, J. E. and LAYNE, C. H. :
Contrasting effects of polycations on
plaquing efficiency of encephalomyocarditis virus variants. J. Virol., 3, 45-51,
1969.

6) DULBECCO, R. and VOGT, M. : Plaque formation and isolation of pure lines with
poliomyelitis viruses. J. Exptl. Med., 99,
167-182, 1954.

7) GREENSTEIN, J. P. and WINITZ, M. : Che-
mistry of the amino acids, vol. 3, p. 1848.
John Wiley and Sons, Inc., New York,
1961.

8) KABUTA, H., YAMAMOTO, S., TANIKAWA, M.
and NAKAGAWA, Y. : Thermoinactivation
of HF and M strains of herpes simplex
virus in various conditions. Kurume
Medical J., 16, 91-99, 1969.

9) KAPLAN, M. M., WICTOR, T. J., MAES, R. F.,
CAMPBELL, J. B. and KOPROWSKI, H. :
Effect of polyions on the infectivity of
rabies virus in tissue culture : Construc-
tion of a single-cycle growth curve. J.
Virol., 1, 145-151, 1967.

10) LOWRY, O. H., ROSEBROUGH, N. J., FARR, A.
L. and RANDALL, R. J. : Protein measure-
ment with the folin phenol reagent. J.
Biol. Chem., 193, 265-275, 1951.

11) NOMURA, S. : Interaction of respiratory
syncytial virus with polyions : Enhancement of infectivity with diethylaminoethyl dextran. Proc. Soc. Exptl. Biol.
Med., 128, 163-166, 1968.

12) PAGANO, J. S. and VAHERI, A. : Enhancement of infectivity of poliovirus RNA
with diethylaminoethyl dextran (DEAE-D).
Arch. Ges. Virus forsch., 17, 456-464, 1965.

13) TILLES, J. G. : Enhancement of interferon
titers by poly-L-ornithine. Proc. Soc.
Exptl. Biol. Med., 125, 996-999, 1967.

14) VOGT, P. K. : Enhancement of cellular
transformation induced by avian sarcoma
viruses. Virology, 33, 175-177, 1967.

15) WALLIS, C. and MELNICK, J. L. : Mechanism
of enhancement of virus plaques by
cationic polymers. J. Virol., 2, 267-274,
1968.

16) YAMAMOTO, S., KABUTA, H. and NAKAGAWA,
Y. : Plaque formation by herpes simplex
viruses in GMK (established grivet monkey kidney) cells. Kurume Medical J., 15,

221-234, 1968.

17) YAMAMOTO, S., KABUTA, H. and NAKAGAWA, Y. : Inhibition of herpes virus adsorption on cells by protamine. Kurume Medical J., **16**, 83-89, 1969.

Persistence of a Repressed Epstein-Barr

Virus Genome in Burkitt Lymphoma Cells

Made Resistant to 5-Bromodeoxyuridine

(thymidine kinase/viral antigen/immunofluorescence/electron microscopy)

BERGE HAMPAR, JEFFERY G. DERGE,

LIDIA M. MARTOS, AND JOHN L. WALKER

ABSTRACT   The P3HR-1 line of human lymphoblastoid cells that is Epstein-Barr virus positive was made resistant to 5-bromodeoxyuridine. Epstein-Barr virus-
associated antigens, but not virus particles, were produced
in P3HR-1(BU) cells maintained on 5-bromodeoxyuridine.
However, virus particles did appear within 4 days after removal of the drug. Thymidine kinase activity was limited
to P3HR-1(BU) cells producing viral antigen, whereas
all control P3HR-1 cells showed thymidine kinase activity
regardless of viral antigen synthesis.
  Cellular DNA in most P3HR-1(BU) cells was made via
pathways that did not involve thymidine kinase. In cells
having a pathway that involved thymidine kinase, a second
DNA of density 1.71 g/cm^2, corresponding to Epstein-
Barr virus, was detected.
  It was concluded that: (a) a repressed Epstein-Barr virus
genome persists in P3HR-1(BU) cells that do not contain
thymidine kinase, with activation of the viral genome
being accompanied by productive infection and the appearance of enzyme, and (b) thymidine kinase activity
in P3HR-1(BU) cells could be used as a marker for viral
genome expression.

Some human lymphoblastoid cell lines show persistent infection with the human Epstein-Barr herpesvirus (EB virus),
which is synthesized in at least a portion of the cell population
at any one time. The persistence of EB virus may be due
either to a low-grade infection with transmission of infectious

Abbreviation: dTK, thymidine kinase; BSS, Hank's balanced
salt solution; PBS, phosphate-buffered saline; SSC, 0.15 M
NaCl–15 mM sodium citrate; P3HR-1(BU) cells, P3HR-1 cells
rendered resistant to BrdU.

virus or to derepression of an integrated viral genome. Cloning experiments with lymphoblastoid cells favor the derepression mechanism (1-3).

The studies reported here concern the properties of EB virus-negative cells in a virus-positive cell population made resistant to 5-bromodeoxyuridine (BrdU). The results indicate that the EB virus genome is maintained in the cells in a repressed or switched-off state, with virus activation being accompanied by productive infection.

MATERIALS AND METHODS

Cells and Media. The EB virus-positive P3HR-1 cell line (4) was propagated as stationary cultures in medium RPMI 1640 containing 20% heat-inactivated fetal calf serum, penicillin, and streptomycin.

Control and experimental cells were checked monthly and found free of pleuropneumonia-like organisms (PPLO) and other contaminants.

Chemicals and Radiochemicals. Aminopterin, Hyp, dT, Ade, and BrdU were obtained from Schwarz/Mann. ATP (disodium) was obtained from B-L Biochemicals. CsCl was obtained from the Harshaw Chemical Co. RNase (beef pancreas 3000 units/mg) was obtained from Worthington Biochemicals.

[methyl-^{3}H]dT (specific activity 6.7 Ci/mmol and 20 Ci/mmol), [6-^{3}H]BrdU (specific activity 26.1 Ci/mmol), [8-^{14}C]Ade (specific activity 51.3 Ci/mol) were obtained from New England Nuclear Corp.

Buffers and Solutions. 90% phenol, redistilled phenol in 10 mmol Tris–1 mmol EDTA–100 mmol NaCl (pH 7.1), 9:1 (v/v); tissue culture medium containing 13.6 μg/ml Hyp–18 ng/ml aminopterin–3.87 μg/ml dT; Tris·maleate, 10 mmol Tris·maleate–150 mmol KCl–20 mmol $MgCl_2$– 1:10,000 2-mercaptoethanol–10 μmol dT (pH 6.4); dTK assay mix, 100 mmol Tris–20 mmol ATP–10 mmol $MgCl_2$– 0.5 MCi [^{3}H]dT (specific activity 20 Ci/mmol) for 10 ml (pH 8.0).

Immunofluorescence and Electron Microscopy. The procedures for the indirect immunofluorescence test and electron microscopy were described (5). EB virus-positive (B-76) and EB virus-negative (B-289) human sera were obtained from Dr. P. Gerber. Fluorescein-conjugated goat antiserum to human globulin was obtained from Huntingdon Research Center, Inc., under Contract NIH69-54 to the National Cancer Institute.

87

Autoradiography. Cells labeled with either [³H]dT or [³H]BrdU were washed with BSS and resuspended in medium containing either dT or BrdU, at a final concentration of 90 µg/ml. The cells were incubated at 37°C for 3 hr, washed with BSS, air dried on slides, and stained for immuno-fluorescence. Coverslips were mounted with 10% glycerin in PBS (v/v); the slides were pressed lightly between the pages of a bibulous paper pad. The cells were scanned by darkfield fluorescence microscopy, and appropriate areas were photographed and their locations were recorded.

The coverslips were removed, the cells were washed in water and air dried. Stripping film (Kodak AR-10) was applied and the slides were exposed for 1–3 weeks at 4°C before developing. The cells were stained for 30 sec in 0.2% crystal violet in 95% methanol (w/v) and the localized areas were scanned under brightfield microscopy.

Incorporation of Isotopes. Cells labeled with appropriate isotopes were washed twice with BSS and once with SSC, resuspended in SSC, and disrupted by sonication. Protein was determined by the method of Lowry *et al.* (6).

Cold 10% Cl_3CCOOH was added to an equal volume of cell sonicate, and precipitates were collected on glass fiber filters for counting in a Beckman LS-133 scintillation counter.

Isopycnic Banding of Labeled DNA. The DNA from cells labeled with appropriate isotopes was isolated by three extractions with 90% phenol (7). The DNA precipitated with ethanol was resuspended in SSC, treated for 30 min at 37°C with 50 µg/ml of RNase (EC 2.7.7.16, heated at 100°C for 10 min), reextracted with 90% phenol, and resuspended in 20 mmol Tris (pH 7.5); CsCl was added to give a starting density of 1.70 g/cm^3. The samples were centrifuged for 72 hr at 20°C in an SW-39 head at 30,000 rpm. Fractions collected with an automatic gradient collector (Instrumentation Specialties Co.) were precipitated with Cl_3CCOOH and collected on glass fiber filters for liquid scintillation counting. Densities were determined by refractometry.

Thymidine Kinase (dTK) Assay. dTK enzyme was assayed by the method of Breitman (8). Cells were washed three times in PBS and resuspended in Tris·maleate. After disruption by sonication, the samples were centrifuged at 100,000 × *g* for 40 min. The supernates (50 µl) were reacted with dTK assay-mixture (50 µl) at 35°C for 30 min. The tubes containing the mixture were placed in ice and 20 µmol EDTA (100 µl) was added. Samples (20 µl) were spotted on Whatman DE81 filter discs for counting.

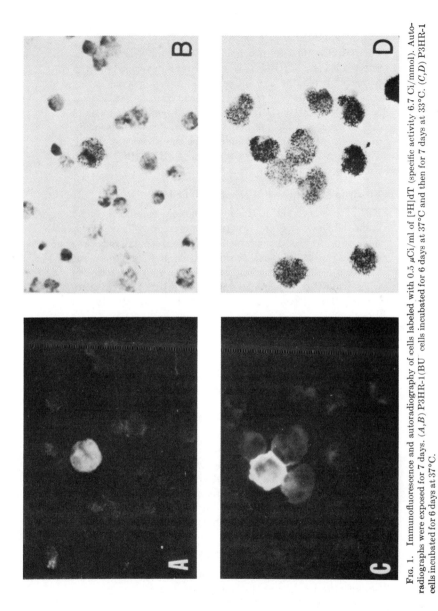

Fig. 1. Immunofluorescence and autoradiography of cells labeled with 0.5 µCi/ml of [³H]dT (specific activity 6.7 Ci/mmol). Autoradiographs were exposed for 7 days. (A,B) P3HR-1(BU cells incubated for 6 days at 37°C and then for 7 days at 33°C. (C,D) P3HR-1 cells incubated for 6 days at 37°C.

RESULTS

BrdU-resistant P3HR-1 cells

P3HR-1 cells that are resistant to 100 μg/ml of BrdU, to be referred to as P3HR-1(BU) cells, were developed over a period of 6 months. No difference in the properties of the cells was noted at drug concentrations of 30 μg/ml and higher. As expected, P3HR-1(BU) cells could not replicate in medium containing hypoxanthine–aminopterin–dT, even when maintained for periods up to 2 months in the absence of BrdU. This suggests a low reversion rate of P3HR-1(BU) cells to BrdU susceptibility.

EB virus replication in P3Hr 1 (BU) cells

EB virus-associated antigen production was studied by immunofluorescence and electron microscopy (Table 1) in replicating and stationary cells (9). Cells containing virus particles (mostly capsids), as well as cells showing herpesvirus "fingerprints" (10), characterized by marginated chromatin with a mottled appearance and reduplicated nuclear membranes, but without particles, were detected by electron microscopy.

Fluorescent-antibody staining in P3HR-1 cells was bright, but the intensity of staining was decreased by 4 days after the addition of BrdU. Low intensity fluorescence was noted in P3HR-1(BU) cells maintained on BrdU, whereas bright fluorescence was apparent within 4 days after removal of the drug.

Ferritin tagging of EB virus capsids (5, 11) was observed in both P3HR-1 and P3HR-1(BU) cells with conjugated human and rabbit antisera to EB virus. Ferritin tagging was also observed in cells showing viral "fingerprints".

We concluded from these studies that: (a) EB virus-associated antigens, but not virus particles, are produced in P3HR-1(BU) cells maintained on 100 μg/ml of BrdU; (b) virus particles appear in P3HR-1(BU) cells within 4 days after removal of the drug.

Thymidine kinase in P3HR-1(BU) cells

Resistance to BrdU should be accompanied by a loss in dTK activity, and a loss in the cell's ability to incorporate exogenous dT or BrdU into DNA (12). This was tested in P3HR-1(BU) cells (Table 2).

Low activity of dTK (5–8% of the activity found in P3HR-1 cells), and little incorporation of [³H]dT and [³H]BrdU (<1% of the levels found in P3HR-1 cells) were noted consistently in P3HR-1(BU) cells, and the levels of incorporation did not increase significantly when cells were maintained for periods of 1–3 months in the absence of BrdU.

90

TABLE 1. *Production of EB virus–associated antigens and virus particles by immunofluorescence (FA) and electron microscopy (EM) in P3HR-1 and P3HR-1(BU) cells in the presence and absence of BrdU**

		Cells					
		P3HR-1			P3HR-1(BU)†		
			% EM +¶			% EM +¶	
Day	BrdU‡	% FA +§	Particles	Fingerprints	% FA +§	Particles	Fingerprints
0	No	3	1	4	3	—	1
	Yes						
4	No	2	1	2	5	1	3
	Yes	3	—	2	3	—	1
7	No	5	4	3	6	3	8
	Yes	2	—	4	5	—	6
Cells transferred to 33°C							
14	No	8	5	2	10	10	2
	Yes	2	—	1	4	—	5

(+) Positive; (−) Negative.

* 5×10^5 cells/ml, incubated at 37°C, were transferred to 33°C on day 7. Cells were tested on days indicated.

† Cells washed at start to remove residual BrdU.

‡ BrdU at a concentration of 100 µg/ml was added at start of experiment. At this concentration, replication of P3HR-1, but not P3HR-1(BU) cells, was inhibited.

§ At least 10^4 cells were screened by FA at each time interval. Intensity of staining in cells treated with BrdUrd was significantly less than in untreated cells.

¶ At least 800 cell profiles on 3 different grids were screened by EM at each time interval.

Relationship between EB virus production and thymidine kinase activity in P3HR-1(BU) cells

The finding of dTK in P3HR-1(BU) cells prompted studies to determine: (a) the proportion of the cell population expressing enzyme, and (b) the relationship, if any, between dTK activity and EB virus production.

P3HR-1 and P3HR-1(BU) cells labeled with either [³H]dT or [³H]BrdU were tested by immunofluorescence and autoradiography. The concentration of [³H]BrdU used (55.9 ng/ml) did not inhibit EB virus replication in either cell line.

Table 3 summarizes the results from one of four reproducible experiments. By 5 days after the addition of either isotope, all of the cells that contained fluorescent antibody in both cultures showed radioactive grains; however, after 12 days in the presence of either isotope, >85% of P3HR-1 cells showed isotope incorporation while isotope incorporation was not seen in P3HR-1(BU) cells that did not contain fluorescent antibody (Fig. 1).

We concluded from these studies that: (a) all virus-producing (fluorescent antibody positive) P3HR-1 and P3HR-1(BU) cells show dTK activity; (b) essentially all P3HR-1 cells show dTK activity regardless of whether virus synthesis occurs; (c) dTK activity in P3HR-1(BU) cells is limited to cells producing viral antigen; and (d) DNA synthesis may precede the appearance of viral antigen by several days.

TABLE 2. *Thymidine kinase (dTK), cell replication, and detection of EB virus-associated antigen production by immunofluorescence (FA) in P3HR-1 and P3HR-1(BU) cells**

		Cells				
		P3HR-1			P3HR-1(BU)†	
		Cell no.§			Cell no.§	
Day	TK‡	× 10⁻⁵	% FA +	TK‡	× 10⁻⁵	% FA +
0	NT	5.0 (86)	1	NT	5.1 (85)	0.5
3	680	6.0 (85)	2	40	5.8 (79)	3
4	860	7.1 (92)	2	50	6.4 (84)	3
7	830	12.2 (89)	4	58	9.3 (88)	5

(NT) Not tested; (+) Positive.

* Cells incubated at 37°C in the absence of BrdU were transferred to 33°C on day 7.

† Cells were washed at start to remove residual BrdU.

‡ nmol of dTMP formed per mg of protein in 100,000 × g cell extract during 30 min at 35°C.

§ Viable cells per ml. Percent viability in parentheses.

92

TABLE 3. *Detection of incorporation of [³H]dT and [³H]BrdU by autoradiography, and of EB virus-associated antigen synthesis by immunofluorescence (FA) in P3HR-1 and P3HR-1(BU) cells**

		Number of cells observed									
		[³H]dT					[³H]BrdU				
		FA+		FA−			FA+		FA−		
Days on Isotope	Cells	³H+	³H−	³H+	³H−	Total	³H+	³H−	³H+	³H−	Total
2	P3HR-1	20	20	114	36	190	23	27	171	31	252
	P3HR-1(BU)	16	26	2	251	295	21	28	0	215	264
5	P3HR-1	23	0	394	86	503	34	0	152	24	210
	P3HR-1(BU)	50	0	2	978	1030	36	0	0	267	303
Cells transferred to 33°C											
12	P3HR-1	28	0	317	22	367	48	0	NT		
	P3HR-1(BU)	58	0	0	572	630	0	0	0	200	248

(NT) Not Tested; (+) Positive; (−) Negative.

* 5 × 10⁵ cells/ml incubated at 37°C were transferred to 33°C on day 7. P3HR-1(BU) cells were washed at start for the removal of residual BrdU. On day 2, either [³H]dT (specific activity 6.7 Ci/mmol) or [³H]BrdU (specific activity 26.1 Ci/mmol) was added at a concentration of 0.5 μCi/ml. Cells were processed for FA and autoradiography on days indicated.

93

Characterization of DNA made in P3HR-1(BU) cells

The finding that dTK activity in P3HR-1(BU) cells was limited to cells producing viral antigen prompted studies to characterize the DNA made in these cells. Since the synthesis of dT by cells does not require dTK, while the utilization of exogenous dT (or BrdU) is dependent upon dTK, cells were grown in the presence of both [^{14}C]Ade and [^{3}H]dT. [^{14}C]Ade is incorporated into DNA made by either dTK-positive or dTK-negative pathways, whereas [^{3}H]dT incorporation is limited to the dTK-positive pathway. As a control, human diploid fibroblast (WI-38) cells were labeled with [^{3}H]dT. The DNA from these cells was isolated and banded in CsCl (Fig. 2).

The ^{3}H-labeled DNA from WI-38 cells (Fig. 2A) banded at a density of 1.69 g/cm^{3}, the density of human DNA. The [^{14}C]Ade- and [^{3}H]dT-labeled DNA from P3HR-1 cells (Fig. 2B) also banded in a single peak at a density of 1.69 g/cm^{3}, with the ratio of [^{14}C]Ade counts to [^{3}H]dT counts (0.15) remaining constant throughout the peak. In contrast, the DNA from P3HR-1(BU) cells (including cells maintained for 2 months in the absence of BrdU) showed two distinct radioactive peaks (Fig. 2C). The ratio of [^{14}C]Ade counts to [^{3}H]dT counts was 325 in the major peak (density 1.69 g/cm^{3}), which corresponded to human DNA, and 9 in the minor peak, which banded at a density of 1.71 g/cm^{3}, corresponding to that of EB virus DNA (13, 14). The absence of a detectable radioactive "viral" DNA peak from P3HR-1 cells (Fig. 2B), which are known to make virus, was apparently due to masking by the preponderant cellular DNA that incorporated [^{3}H]dT.

We concluded from these studies that: (a) cellular DNA (1.69 g/cm^{3}) synthesis in all P3HR-1 cells utilizes both dTK-positive and dTK-negative pathways; (b) cellular DNA synthesis in some P3HR-1(BU) cells utilizes only dTK-negative pathways, while DNA synthesis in other cells utilizes both dTK-positive and negative pathways, and (c) "viral" DNA (1.71 g/cm^{3}) in P3HR-1(BU) cells is made only in those cells with a dTK-positive pathway.

DISCUSSION

Persistence of a repressed EB virus genome in P3HR-1(BU) cells is concluded from the following observations:

EB virus-particle formation in P3HR-1(BU) cells was inhibited at BrdU concentrations >30 µg/ml, although viral antigen was still synthesized and viral induced cytopathic changes (e.g., "fingerprints") were still apparent. Similar inhibition of infectious virus synthesis by BrdU is seen with other herpesviruses (15); this inhibition may be attributed

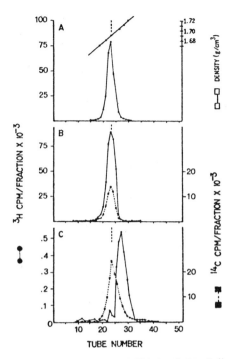

FIG. 2. Isopycnic banding of DNA in CsCl. Cells were incubated for 6 days at 37°C with 2 μCi/ml of [³H]dT (specific activity 20 Ci/mmol) and 0.1 μCi/ml of [¹⁴C]Ade (specific activity 51.3 mCi/mol), as indicated. (*A*) WI-38 cells labeled with [³H]dT. (*B*) P3HR-1 cells labeled simultaneously with [³H]dT and [¹⁴C]Ade. (*C*) P3HR-1(BU) cells labeled simultaneously with [³H]dT and [¹⁴C]Ade.

to faulty transcription of viral DNA in regions where BrdU has been incorporated (16). The incorporation of BrdU into P3HR-1(BU) cells was demonstrated. Since P3HR-1(BU) cells have been maintained for over 8 months in the continued presence of BrdU concentrations >30 μg/ml, and since complete EB virus synthesis is evident shortly after removal of the drug, we conclude that the persistence of a chronic EB virus infection in P3HR-1(BU) cells was not due to transmission of infectious virus.

The dTK activity seen in P3HR-1(BU) cells was related, apparently, to the continued presence of the EB virus genome, since enzyme activity was restricted to cells producing viral antigen. Although the mechanism by which P3HR-1(BU) cells spontaneously converted from a dTK-negative to a dTK-positive state with concomitant viral antigen synthesis has yet to be elucidated, three possibilities may be considered.

First, cell-to-cell transmission of complete or incomplete

EB virus particles induced enzyme in dTK-negative cells. This would be similar to dTK induction seen with cells infected by herpes simplex virus (17). Transmission of infectious EB virus with resultant dTK induction may be excluded (*vide supra*). Transmission of incomplete EB virus particles with resultant dTK induction may also be excluded, since viral antigen and "viral" DNA synthesis were seen only in dTK-positive cells. Persistence of an unmodified viral genome under conditions where BrdU was continuously being incorporated into DNA would seem untenable, based on the known mutagenic effects of this drug. The only plausible way in which an infectious herpesvirus could persist in the continued presence of BrdU would be by a mutation that converted the virus to a dTK-negative state, whereby the drug could no longer be incorporated into viral DNA. This would be analogous to the BrdU-induced dTK-negative strains of herpes simplex virus (18). If transmission of dTK-negative EB virus mutants was responsible for the persistent infection, we should have seen viral antigen synthesis in dTK-negative cells.

The second possibility is that the EB virus genome persisted in dTK-negative P3HR-1(BU) cells in a repressed state, with cell-coded dTK being activated concomitant with virus activation. This possibility assumes that the cell's resistance to BrdU was due to a mutation affecting enzyme expression rather than the loss of a structural gene. Under these conditions, the expression of cellular dTK would probably have to be under control of the viral genome, since dTK was not being expressed in the absence of viral-antigen synthesis. Although the likelihood that these sequence of events were occurring in P3HR-1(BU) cells seems remote, it cannot be definitively excluded.

The third possibility is that the EB virus genome persisted in dTK-negative P3HR-1(BU) cells in a repressed state, with viral-coded dTK being activated concomitant with virus activation. This possibility assumes that the cell's resistance to BrdU was due to a mutation resulting either in permanent loss or permanent suppression of the cell's structural gene coding for dTK, without affecting the structural gene coding for viral dTK. Although final proof must await results of experiments to determine the origin of the dTK being expressed in P3HR-1(BU) cells, two factors make this third possibility particularly attractive. First, a completely repressed viral genome would not express any gene functions, including dTK. Second, a viral-dTK structural gene that is repressed would not be subjected to the same selective pressures in the presence of BrdU as would be a cellular–dTK structural gene that was being expressed.

We believe that the findings reported here justify the conclusion that a human herpesvirus, in this case EB virus, can indeed persist in a human cell in a completely repressed state. Additional evidence for this conclusion has now been obtained and will be reported separately (19). This involves drug-induced activation of the EB virus genome in long-term cultures of "virus-negative" human lymphoblastoid cells.

We thank Mrs. M. A. Burroughs, Mrs. M. Tagamets, Miss S. Birkhead, Miss C. Owen, Mrs. D. Krell, Mr. M. Chakrabarty, and Mr. D. Simms for technical assistance. This work was supported in part by Contract NIH71-2097 from the Special Virus-Cancer Program, National Cancer Institute, National Institutes of Health, Bethesda, Md. 20014.

1. Hinuma, Y., and J. T. Grace, Jr., *Cancer*, **22**, 1089 (1968).
2. Maurer, B. A., T. Imamura, and S. M. Wilbert, *Cancer Res.*, **30**, 2870 (1970).
3. Miller, M. H., D. Stitt, and G. Miller, *J. Virol.*, **6**, 699 (1970).
4. Hinuma, Y., M. Konn, J. Yamaguchi, D. J. Wudarski, J. R. Blakeslee, Jr., and J. T. Grace, Jr., *J. Virol*, **1**, 1045 (1967).
5. Hampar, B., P. Gerber, K. C. Hsu, L. M. Martos, J. L. Walker, R. F. Siguenza, and G. A. Wells, *J. Nat. Cancer Inst.*, **45**, 75 (1970).
6. Lowry, O. H., N. J. Rosebrough, L. Farr, and R. J. Randall, *J. Biol. Chem.*, **193**, 265 (1951).
7. Marmur, J., *J. Mol. Biol.*, **3**, 208 (1901).
8. Breitman, T. R., *Biochim. Biophys. Acta.*, **67**, 153 (1963).
9. Hinuma, Y., M. Konn, J. Yamaguchi, and J. T. Grace, Jr., *J. Virol.*, **1**, 1203 (1967).
10. Nii, S., C. Morgan, and H. M. Rose, *J. Virol.*, **2**, 517 (1968).
11. Hampar, B., K. C. Hsu, L. M. Martos, and J. L. Walker, *Proc. Nat. Acad. Sci. USA*, **68**, 1407 (1971).
12. Kit, S., D. R. Dubbs, L. J. Piekarski, and T. C. Hsu, *Exp. Cell Res.*, **31**, 297 (1963).
13. Schulte-Holthausen, H., and H. Zur Hausen, *Virology*, **40**, 776 (1970).
14. Wagner, E. K., B. Roizman, T. Savage, P. G. Spear, M. Mizell, F. E. Durr, and D. Sypowicz, *Virology*, **42**, 257 (1970).
15. Siminoff, P., *Virology*, **24**, 1 (1964).
16. Kaplan, A. S., T. Ben-Porat, and T. Kamiya, *Ann. N.Y. Acad. Sci.*, **130**, 226 (1965).
17. Kit, S., and D. R. Dubbs, *Biochem. Biophys, Res. Commun.*, **11**, 55 (1963).
18. Kit, S., and D. R. Dubbs, *Biochem. Biophys. Res. Commun.*, **13**, 500 (1963).
19. Hampar, B., J. G. Derge, L. M. Martos, and J. L. Walker, *Proc. Nat. Acad. Sci. USA.*, **69** (1972), in press.

Clinical Evaluation of Kethoxal

Against Cutaneous Herpes Simplex

G. E. UNDERWOOD AND F. R. NICHOL

A 2.5% preparation of kethoxal in cream was compared with the cream placebo for efficacy against cutaneous herpes simplex in a double-blind clinical study. The kethoxal formulation was not significantly more effective than the placebo. This conclusion was based on subjective impressions of the patients, observations by the physicians, and quantitative measurement of herpesvirus recovered from the lesions. It was suggested that the lack of clinical activity, in contrast to the marked activity against experimental infections in laboratory animals, resulted from the fact that high levels of herpesvirus were already present in the skin before symptoms were noted.

Kethoxal demonstrated outstanding activity when applied topically to cutaneous herpes simplex lesions on experimental animals (4). The compound, 3-ethoxy-2-oxobutyraldehyde hydrate, seemed a promising candidate for evaluation against "cold sores" in man. Animal toxicology studies indicated that it was safe to proceed with human topical tolerance testing. Phase 1 evaluation in prison volunteers demonstrated that a 2.5% concentration of the formulated drug was well tolerated topically. Studies examining efficacy against cutaneous herpes in man were then initiated in cooperation with four investigators. This report describes the clinical procedures and summarizes the results obtained in the efficacy study. Clinical results are further discussed in relation to controlled studies with an experimental cutaneous herpes infection in hairless mice and response of this laboratory infection to kethoxal treatment.

MATERIALS AND METHODS

General clinical procedure. Only adults with a history of recurrent cutaneous herpes simplex were accepted for the study. Each volunteer was given a coded tube containing drug or placebo, a list of instructions, and a form to be completed at the time of his next herpes episode. At the first symptoms of an incipient cold sore, the patient started treatment. He also visited the physician on day 1 for physical examination, attempted virus isolation, and blood sampling. The patient visited the physician again on days 2 and 3 for physical examination and attempted virus isolation. A post-treatment blood sample was obtained on day 3. The patient visited the physician for his final checkup 1 week after the first symptoms were noted.

Treatment procedure. On the form provided, the patient recorded the time when he first noted symptoms of a new cold sore. Symptoms were described by checking appropriate boxes on the form, i.e., tingling, itching, burning, pain, redness, swelling, blisters, oozing, soft scab, and dry crust. Topical treatment was started immediately, with the contents of the coded tube which contained either 2.5% kethoxal in cream or the cream alone (placebo). Self-treatment was administered every 2 hr up to a maximum of five treatments on day 1 and an additional four times at 3- to 4-hr intervals on day 2, at which time treatment was terminated.

Virus isolations. The physician examined the lesion at the time of each patient visit and recorded his findings on the appropriate form supplied to him. He also took samples for attempted virus isolation on days 1, 2, and 3 by gently swabbing the lesion with a sterile swab moistened with cell culture medium. The swab was broken off into a small serum bottle containing medium and stored immediately at -20 C. Muller's samples were assayed by E. C. Herrmann of the Mayo Clinic. All other virus isolates were sent to The Upjohn Co. and were assayed by the procedure described below.

Each sample was tested for herpes simplex virus (HSV) by inoculating 0.2 ml into each of two rabbit kidney tubes. One blind passage was made 5 to 6 days postinoculation from tubes showing no cytopathology. Fluids were harvested from positive tubes after disrupting the cells by freezing, and a sample was mixed with an equal volume of HSV immune serum prepared in rabbits. The original lesion swab samples from which confirmed HSV was isolated were then titrated by plaque assay on tissue culture dishes containing a monolayer of primary rabbit kidney cells. Two dishes were used for each 10-fold dilution and titers were calculated as plaque-forming units (PFU) per milliliter of swab sample.

Investigators. The cooperating physicians and the number of usable case reports submitted by each were: R. D. Carr, Ohio State University, Columbus, 8 cases; S. A. Muller, Mayo Clinic, Rochester, Minn., 18 cases; W. A. Rye, The Upjohn Co., Kalamazoo, Mich., 85 cases; R. H. Grekin and P. W. Wang, Kalamazoo, Mich., 62 cases.

Blood studies. Hematocrit, hemoglobin, total white count, differential, serum glutamic oxalacetic

99

TABLE 1. *Patient profile*

Patient data	Kethoxal	Placebo
Number................	58	65
Age (mean year).......	37	38
Sex (females)..........	30 (52)[a]	34 (52)
Race (white)..........	58 (100)	65 (100)

[a] Values in parentheses are percentages.

transaminase, bilirubin, alkaline phosphatase, and creatinine were determined. Values obtained were compared to normal ranges for the respective testing laboratory.

Statistical evaluation of efficacy. The patient recorded the condition of the lesion at the time treatment was started, and the physician rated the lesion on the same scale on days 1, 2, and 3. This description was coded on a six-point scale showing the stage of development as: (i) no signs or symptoms; (ii) tingling, itching, burning, or pain, or all four; (iii) redness or swelling, or both; (iv) blisters; (v) oozing or soft scab, or both; (vi) dry crust. The progress of the lesion was assessed on days 1, 2, and 3 as "better," "same," or "worse," relative to its condition at start of treatment.

Hairless mouse studies. Mice were infected cutaneously with HSV and treated topically with kethoxal, and lesions were scored as previously described (4). In addition, virus yields from the mice were determined by immersing a sterile cotton swab into a 3-ml vial containing 1.5 ml of medium 199 with 5% heat-inactivated fetal calf serum and gently swabbing the affected area. The saturated swabs were broken at the stem, returned to the vials, sealed, and frozen at −55 C before titration in duplicate on primary rabbit kidney monolayers.

RESULTS

Of the 173 complete and usable case reports received from the four investigators, 123 described patients who started treatment within 3 hr of the time that symptoms of an incipient herpes lesion were first noted. Since early treatment should have the best chance of success, the statistical analyses were performed on these 123 case reports. There was no significant difference ($P > 0.05$) between the kethoxal- and placebo-treated groups with respect to age, sex, or race (Table 1). No blood changes due to kethoxal treatment were observed.

Efficacy was evaluated objectively by examining changes in appearance of the lesions as described above. There was no significant difference between the two treatments on any day (Table 2). Benefit of treatment was also assessed by con-

TABLE 2. *Progress of lesion compared to its condition at start of treatment*

Treatment	Better on day			Same on day			Worse on day		
	1	2	3	1	2	3	1	2	3
Kethoxal.......	2 (5)[a]	3 (6)	8 (14)	33 (87)	27 (57)	10 (18)	3 (8)	17 (36)	39 (68)
Placebo........	3 (6)	2 (9)	10 (16)	40 (78)	19 (41)	11 (17)	8 (16)	23 (50)	43 (67)

[a] Values in parentheses expressed as percentages.

TABLE 3. *Evaluation of treatment based on change in virus titers*

Treatment	Very beneficial	Bene-ficial	No effect	Became worse	Much worse
Kethoxal....	2 (7)[a]	11 (39)	3 (11)	7 (25)	5 (18)
Placebo.....	1 (3)	8 (25)	6 (19)	11 (34)	6 (19)

[a] Values in parentheses are expressed as percentages.

TABLE 4. *Isolation of herpesvirus*

Treatment	Herpesvirus present on day		
	1	2	3
Kethoxal....	15 (36)[a]	20 (46)	14 (29)
Placebo.....	17 (35)	23 (55)	17 (30)

[a] Values in parentheses are expressed as percentages.

TABLE 5. *Subjective evaluation of treatment*

Treatment	Benefit obtained				
	Very much	Much	Some	Little	None
Kethoxal....	8 (14)[a]	30 (34)	14 (24)	5 (9)	11 (19)
Placebo.....	11 (17)	25 (38)	12 (20)	3 (5)	13 (20)

[a] Values in parentheses are expressed as percentages.

sidering the change in virus titer with respect to time. In making this evaluation, consideration was given to whether virus titer decreased or increased in successive samples and to the extent of this titer change. Only those cases were included in which more than one swab sample was taken and in which HSV was isolated from at least one of the samples. Assignment of such cases was made to one of the categories listed in Table 3, without knowing whether the patient had received drug or placebo treatment. Obviously, this procedure would not include patients in whom there may have been initial virus present which was eradicated by the treatment for the 3-day sampling period. Such sterilization may have occurred in some patients, but, if so, it was not a consistent response. This can be inferred from Table 3, which indicates that after treatment the virus titer increased in lesions of about half the virus-yielding patients, both in drug- and placebo-treated groups. It is apparent from the data in Table 3 that response of the two treatment groups was not significantly different based on changes in virus titers.

The two groups were compared each day by the chi square test for the number of subjects who had herpes present. All were included who had at least one sample taken for virus isolation. The totals vary from day to day because not all patients were sampled each day. The treatment groups were not significantly different (Table 4).

Each physician was also asked to record on the case report form his estimate of the amount of benefit derived from the treatment. This subjective measure of efficacy showed no significant difference ($P > 0.05$) between the two groups (Table 5). Response to this question was also examined by limiting the cases to those in which herpesvirus was actually found (Table 6). Again, there was no significant difference between the two groups. Lesions at the treatment site developed in equivalent numbers of patients in the two groups (Table 7), and the examining physicians characterized all of these as "typical" herpes simplex lesions.

Mouse studies. Several experiments were performed in hairless mice as an aid to understanding the clinical results. In a typical experiment, 20 mice were infected cutaneously with HSV; no lesions appeared until the 3rd day after virus inoculation. All animals had $2+$ or greater lesion scores on the 4th day after infection, and all animals were dead 1 week postinfection.

Table 8 presents data illustrating the favorable effects of kethoxal application to cutaneously infected hairless mice at different times after HSV inoculation. Excellent protection resulted from a single topical treatment of the infected area with kethoxal at any time between 1 and 6 hr after infection. The most effective time of treatment appeared to be about 4 hr after virus inoculation, as evidenced by lesion development in only 20% of the mice and an average virus yield in those mice developing lesions of less than 1% of that recovered from the controls on the 3rd day postinfection. In addition to prevention of lesion formation in 80% of the mice treated at 4 hr postinfection, it was noted that the lesions completely healed in six of the eight mice which did develop lesions, and these six mice lived for 1 month, at which time the experiment was terminated. Similar recovery occurred with mice treated with kethoxal at 2 hr postinfection, with somewhat smaller percentages recovering in

TABLE 6. *Amount of benefit in those cases in which herpesvirus was found*

| Group | Treatment | Amount of benefit | | | | |
		Very much	Much	Some	Little	None
Lesions	Kethoxal	1 (3)[a]	12 (34)	8 (23)	5 (14)	9 (26)
≤ 3 hr old	Placebo	2 (6)	13 (41)	8 (25)	1 (3)	8 (25)
All lesions	Kethoxal	1 (2)	15 (30)	13 (26)	8 (16)	13 (26)
	Placebo	3 (7)	14 (33)	12 (28)	2 (5)	12 (28)

[a] Values in parentheses are expressed as percentages.

TABLE 7. *Lesion formation at treated site*

Treatment	Yes	No	No response
Kethoxal.....	56 (97)[a]	2 (3)	0 (0)
Placebo..	58 (89)	5 (8)	2 (3)

[a] Values in parentheses are expressed as percentages.

the 1- and 6-hr groups (Table 8).

To determine the length of time kethoxal remained active on hairless mouse skin, groups of 10 mice each were scratched as for virus inoculation and then treated topically with 5% kethoxal in water. Separate groups were again scratched and inoculated with HSV at 15-min intervals thereafter for 1 hr. The results (Table 9) show a rapid loss of activity within 60 min of kethoxal application.

DISCUSSION

This study, as did a previous one with a different compound (5), clearly illustrates how essential placebo-controlled, blind-label procedures are when clinically evaluating an agent against cutaneous HSV. Thus, 72% of the kethoxal-treated patients appeared to derive at least some benefit from the treatment (Table 5), but the comparable figure for the placebo group was 75%, indicating the lack of a drug-related effect. Results obtained in drug-treated and placebo-treated groups were also similar for other parameters studied. and there was no evidence that kethoxal beneficially influenced the course of the infection. Since the compound was outstandingly active against cutaneous HSV infections in the laboratory (4), an explanation was sought for this lack of clinical activity.

The protocol was designed to initiate treatment as early as possible, i.e., when the patient felt the first symptoms of an incipient herpes lesion. Most of the patients started treatment within 3 hr of the time that symptoms were first noted, but over 50% of these patients indicated that their lesions had already progressed to the "blister" or vesicle stage. It would seem, therefore, that in the human disease appreciable virus replication has occurred before any symptoms of an approaching cold sore are noted. The burning, itching, and tingling, which often represent first symptoms, may indeed result from early interaction between viral antigen and its antibody; such antibody is invariably present in the serum of

TABLE 8. *Mice treated topically with a single application of 5% kethoxal in water at various times postinfection (PI) with herpesvirus (HSV)*

Treatment		No. of mice	No. with lesion scores ≥ 2 on day			Avg titer[a] on day 3 PI	No. of mice that recovered
Compound	Time (hr) PI		4	6	8		
Kethoxal	1	40	ND	15	15 (38)[c]	3.7	9/15
	2	40	2	11	11 (28)	3.2	9/11
	4	40	2	8	8 (20)	2.8	6/8
	6	40	ND	19	19 (48)	ND	9/19
	8	40	ND	30	30 (75)	3.2	ND
	10	10	4	7	7 (70)	4.8	ND
Control		60	60	60	60 (100)	5.4	0/60

[a] Expressed as $\log_{10}$ PFU/0.5 ml of HSV in swab sample.
[b] Not determined.
[c] Values in parentheses are expressed as percentages.

TABLE 9. *Duration of anti-herpesvirus activity of 5% kethoxal in water on hairless mouse skin*

Time of treatment (min before infection)	No. of mice	No. with lesion scores ≥ 2 on day 6
15	10	1
30	10	3
45	10	7
60	10	9
Control	10	10

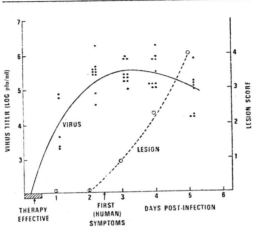

FIG. 1. *Cutaneous herpesvirus on hairless mice. Virus: each • represents the virus titer for an individual mouse. Titers less than 10² PFU/ml caused fewer than 10 points on days 1 and 5.*

individuals who suffer from recurrent herpes lesions.

We can now consider, for purposes of comparison, the results obtained with experimental cutaneous herpes in hairless mice. If we plot on a single graph levels of virus recoverable from the inoculated area, "lesion score," and interval during which kethoxal therapy is effective, we find the interesting relationships shown in Fig. 1. These hairless mouse data suggest that it would be very unlikely that kethoxal treatment would be efficacious if it were delayed until first symptoms occur. In the hairless mouse, there is no sign of a lesion at 48 hr after virus inoculation, but most of the mice will have tiny vesicles at 72 hr post-infection, by which time the virus titer has reached its maximum. If the situation is comparable to man, there would probably be no symptoms of an impending lesion until at least 60 hr post-infection, i.e., shortly before the appearance of lesions. Kethoxal treatment is not effective in hairless mice, however, if delayed more than 10 to 12 hr after virus is inoculated.

It is not possible to establish direct correlations in a single host with respect to time of infection, appearance of first symptoms, and interval of effective therapy because, on the one hand, one cannot ethically infect volunteers with herpes virus and, on the other hand, one cannot question mice regarding their symptoms. The various human and mouse results taken together, however, indicate that virus titer in the cells is near maximum by the time symptoms are noted and that this is too late for treatment with kethoxal to have a beneficial effect on the course of the lesion. In fact, it appears unlikely that therapy with any antiviral agent would be effective in curing such a lesion; perhaps the most that could be expected is that a drug might prevent spread and development of new lesions. Of course, the great majority of recurrent herpes lesions are self-limiting and do not spread even without therapy.

Various agents have been claimed to be effective in treatment of cold sores, but none is yet accepted as possessing well established activity. The most thoroughly studied compound is 5-iodo-2'-deoxyuridine (IDU), but even here the clinical results are conflicting. MacCallum and Juel-Jensen reported activity with 5% IDU in dimethyl sulfoxide (DMSO) in a double-blind trial involving 16 patients (2). Average duration of the attack was reportedly reduced 64% in the IDU-treated group, but it was reduced 43% in those treated with DMSO only, indicating that the solvent alone was about two-thirds as effective as the drug-in-solvent in this rather small group of patients. Turnbull et al. also reported highly favorable results with topical IDU by using a 1% solution in DMSO (3), but these tests were uncontrolled and, therefore, suffer from the severe limitations imposed by the "placebo effect" noted earlier.

Kibrick and Katz, on the other hand, in a double-blind controlled study involving a total of more than 150 cases of herpetic lesions of the face, found no evidence that topically applied IDU was more beneficial than was placebo (1). In separate studies, they used 0.5% IDU in ointment and 0.1% IDU in 1.4% polyvinyl alcohol solution. IDU was ineffective in both studies, even when those cases in which treatment was initiated within 12 hr of onset were considered separately. Because of the disparaties in results obtained in these and other IDU studies, it is as yet impossible to arrive at any final conclusion concerning its efficacy against cutaneous HSV. Adequately controlled clinical data are not yet available for making valid judgments on other agents with claimed activity.

ACKNOWLEDGMENTS

Numerous persons contributed to the successful completion of this study. Some were mentioned previously in this report and a few of the others are listed here. L. E. Rhuland and C. A Schlagel contributed useful suggestions concerning design of the protocol. W. A. Rye and his staff in Industrial Health made possible the participation of Upjohn volunteers in the study. The Upjohn Clinical Research Laboratory, directed by J. T. Sobota, assayed blood samples submitted by Drs. Grekin and Wang. S. D. Weed provided technical assistance in the human studies, and R. D. Hamilton typed and titrated the clinical virus isolates. Special appreciation is expressed to Marie H. Maile who, with the technical assistance of D. W. Johnson, analyzed the data and interpreted the statistical results. The contribution of each of these individuals to the success of the study is gratefully acknowledged.

LITERATURE CITED

1. Kibrick, S., and A. S. Katz. 1970. Topical idoxuridine in recurrent herpes simplex. Ann. N.Y. Acad. Sci. 173:83–89.
2. MacCallum, F. O., and D. C. Juel Jensen. 1966. Herpes simplex virus skin infection in man treated with idoxuridine in dimethyl sulfoxide. Results of double-blind controlled trial. Brit. Med. J. 2:805–807.
3. Turnbull, B. C., I. MacGregor, and H. C. W. Stringer. 1969. The enhancing effect of dimethylsulfoxide vehicle upon the anti-viral actions of 5-iododeoxyuridine. N. Z. Med. J. 70:317–320.
4. Underwood, G. E. 1968. Kethoxal for treatment of cutaneous herpes simplex. Proc. Soc. Exp. Biol. Med. 129:235–239.
5. Underwood, G. E. 1970. Clinical evaluation of 4'-[2-nitro-1-(p-tolylthio)ethyl] acetanilide (U-3243) against cutaneous herpes simplex. Ann. N.Y. Acad. Sci. 173:782–793.

Herpesvirus Saimiri: *In Vitro* Sensitivity to Virus-Induced Interferon and to Polyriboinosinic Acid:Polyribocytidylic Acid[1] (35451)

H. H. BARAHONA AND L. V. MELENDEZ

Virus-induced interferon and the synthetic double-stranded RNA, polyriboinosinic acid:polyribocytidylic acid (Poly I:C) have been shown to inhibit the growth of some members of the herpesviruses group (1–6). Interferon and Poly I:C have also been shown to inhibit the growth of tumors produced by viruses in mice and hamsters, as well as other tumors induced by chemical carcinogens or tumors not known to contain infectious oncogenic viruses (7–9).

Previous studies from this laboratory (10, 11) reported the isolation of a herpesvirus (H. saimiri) from the squirrel monkey (*Saimiri sciureus*) which is capable of inducing a malignant lymphoma of the reticulum cell type in nonhuman primates and in rabbits.

This report deals with the induction of resistance against H. saimiri in owl monkey kidney cultures treated with Newcastle disease virus (NDV) interferon or with Poly I:C. The significance of these findings is discussed.

Materials and Methods. Cells. Primary and continuous cultures of owl monkey kidney (OMK) were grown as monolayers on plastic

[1] This investigation was supported by NIH, U.S. Public Health Service Grant No. RR 00168-09.

250-ml flasks (Falcon) with 15 ml of Eagle's minimum essential medium containing 10% fetal calf serum (MEM-10). Full grown monolayers were maintained in the same medium. For virus titration and virus plaque-inhibition assay of interferon the cells were transferred into 35- and 60-mm plastic dishes and kept at 37° in a 5% CO_2 atmosphere. Penicillin and streptomycin were added to all media employed in this work, at a concentration of 250 units/ml, and 250 μg/ml, respectively. OMK cultures at least 2-months-old were employed in these studies to avoid interference due to the presence of indigenous viruses.

Viruses. H. saimiri strain S-295C was used in these studies. Stocks were prepared and assayed in OMK cells. Vesicular stomatitis virus (VSV), strain New Jersey, was obtained from Dr. R. P. Hanson, The University of Wisconsin, Madison. Stocks were prepared in rabbit kidney primary cultures (RKP) and assayed in RKP and OMK cells. NDV, strain Kansas-Manhattan, was obtained from the same source and stock pools were grown and assayed in the allantoic chamber of 10-day-old embryonated eggs.

Virus titrations and plaque assay. The infectivity assay (ID_{50}) was carried out in triplicate 35-mm dishes. The plaque assay method and the agar overlay medium employed have been described elsewhere (12). The PFU determinations were done in 60-mm dishes and for counting of the plaques, the monolayers were stained with 1% gentian violet in 20% alcohol.

Preparation and assay of interferon. Stock owl monkey interferon (OM-IF) was prepared following a procedure described previously (13). Confluent OMK cultures were infected with NDV at a m.o.i. of approximately 3 PFU/cell and incubated in a 5% CO_2 atmosphere for 18–19 hr. To rid the interferon-containing medium of residual virus, the tissue culture fluids were centrifuged at 100,000g and dialyzed against large volumes of 0.03–0.1 M HCl (pH 2.0) followed by dialysis in buffered saline solution containing phenol red (pH 7.2). Interferon samples were stored at −20° and assayed by the plaque-inhibition technique with approximately 50–80 PFU of VSV.

The end point of the titration was expressed as that dilution of interferon in which the plaque number was reduced to 50% compared with the control count. The stocks of owl monkey interferon prepared had a titer of 1:1000 per 3 ml. Other characteristics of this interferon were its acid stability, species specificity, failure to sediment at 10,000g for 1.5 hr, and heat stability.

Reagents. Poly I:C was purchased from Microbiological Associates, Bethesda, Maryland, in concentrations of 1 mg/ml. Each lot used was tested for its ability to protect OMK cells against 50 to 80 PFU of VSV. In every test, significative protection (50% plaque reduction) was obtained at concentrations of 0.1 to 0.01 μg/ml after a pretreatment time of 5–6 hr. Diethylaminoethyl-dextran (DEAE-D) from Pharmacia, Uppsala, Sweden, was prepared as a 1% solution in demineralized water, autoclaved for 10 min at 121° and stored at 4°.

Results. Expt. 1. Sensitivity to NDV-induced interferon. The sensitivity of H. saimiri to the effect of interferon was tested in OMK cultures grown in 35-mm dishes pretreated for 6 hr with 2 ml of a dilution 1:16 of OM-IF in Eagle's basal medium with 0.5% fetal calf serum (BME-0.5). After withdrawing the interferon medium the cultures were challenged with serial tenfold dilutions of H. saimiri, incubated for 1 hr at 37°, and overlaid with 2 ml of MEM-10. A second group of similarly treated cultures were overlaid with 2 ml of a dilution 1:16 of OM-IF and this was kept for the duration of the experiment. Untreated control dishes were also infected. Results presented in Fig. 1 indicate that in the first group of OM-IF-treated cultures (6 hr pretreatment alone) there was a delay of 24–48 hr in the onset of cytopathic effect (CPE). The onset of CPE was even further delayed (6 to 7 days) in the second group of cultures kept in OM-IF

112

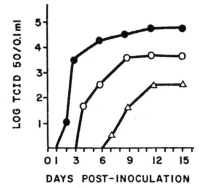

FIG. 1. Cytopathic effect of H. saimiri ($\log_{10}$ TCID$_{50}$) in OMK cultures: (O) cells treated with interferon for 6 hr before inoculation; (△) cells treated as the previous group and maintained with interferon after inoculation; (●) untreated control cultures.

after infection. Furthermore, the degree of the CPE was reduced in both groups of interferon-treated cells when compared with the nontreated infected controls. By the 12th day after infection there was no more increase in virus titers in any of the three infected groups of cultures. The end-point titration indicated differences of approximately 1 and 2 logs in titer in cultures pretreated for 6 hr and in cultures kept in interferon medium for the duration of the experiment, respectively.

Expt. 2. Action of Poly I:C on H. saimiri multiplication. Several concentrations of Poly I:C in BME-0.5 ranging from 20 to 0.001 μg/ml were added to groups of different sets of OMK cultures. These were then incubated for 6 hr at 37° in a CO_2 incubator. Thereafter the monolayers were washed twice with 5 ml of BME-0.5 and infected with serial tenfold dilutions of H. saimiri. After an incubation period of 1 hr, the cultures were overlaid with agar medium and the plaques were counted 10–12 days later.

Pretreatment of the cultures with the polynucleotide at concentrations of 10 and 20 μg/ml gave approximately 1 log protection (81% inhibition) when compared with titrations done in untreated cultures (Table I). However, with 10 μg/ml there were occasion-

113

TABLE I. Inhibition of H. saimiri Multiplication in OMK Cultures by Poly I:C.

Poly I:C (μg/ml)	H. saimiri titer (PFU/0.1 ml)	Inhibition (%)
20	4.5×10^4	81.0
10	4.0×10^4	83.5
1	2.0×10^5	16.6
0.1	2.1×10^5	12.5
0.01	2.3×10^5	4.2
0.001	1.9×10^5	20.0
0.0 (control)	2.4×10^5	—

al experiments in which protection was not constant. However, Poly I:C at a concentration of 20 μg/ml always gave a constant level of protection.

Expt. 3. Effect of DEAE-D on the protective activity of Poly I:C. Previous reports which indicate that the protective activity of polynucleotides could be enhanced by the presence of polycation DEAE-D (14, 15) led us to study its effect on OMK cultures infected with H. saimiri. These experiments were conducted in the same way as Expt. 2, with the difference that a group of cultures were pretreated for 6 hr with a medium containing 50 μg/ml of DEAE-D and varying concentrations of Poly I:C. As shown in Table II, the protective activity of Poly I:C at 10 and 20 μg/ml was considerably increased by the addition of the polycation. The size of the plaques was also reduced. This enhancing activity was not observed when DEAE-D was added to polynucleotide concentrations lower than 10 μg/ml. The polycation as the only additive in the medium failed to induce resistance of H. saimiri infection, and did not have toxic effect on the OMK cell cultures.

Expt. 4. Effect of Poly I:C plus DEAE-D added 1 hr after the infection of the cells. To evaluate further the activity of the polycation as an enhancer of the protective effect of Poly I:C, OMK cultures were infected with tenfold dilutions of H. saimiri and, after an incubation period of 1 hr for

114

TABLE II. Enhancement of Poly I:C Inhibition of H. saimiri Multiplication in OMK Cultures by DEAE-D.

Poly I:C (μg/ml)	DEAE-D (μg/ml)	H. saimiri titer (PFU/0.1 ml)	Inhibition (%)
20	0	1.2×10^4	94.0
10	0	3.5×10^4	82.5
1	0	1.4×10^5	30.0
20	50	3.0×10^2	99.9
10	50	6.3×10^2	99.7
1	50	1.6×10^5	20.0
0.1	50	4.5×10^5	0.0
0	50	2.4×10^5	0.0
0	0 (control)	2.0×10^5	—

virus adsorption, the cells were treated for 6 hr with Poly I:C at various concentrations, and with Poly I:C and DEAE-D.

The results presented in Table III show that when the cells were treated with the polynucleotide alone at concentrations of 40, 20, and 10 μg/ml, there was an induction of resistance against H. saimiri similar to the one observed in Expts. 2 and 3 in which the cells were treated with Poly I:C for 6 hr previous to the challenge with the virus. However, the resistance induced in cells pre-inoculated with the virus and then exposed to similar varying concentrations of the ribonucleotide was considerably enhanced by the inclusion in the inducer medium of 50 μg/ml of DEAE-D. When Poly I:C at concentrations of 40 and 20 μg/ml plus DEAE-D at the concentration previously indicated were used together, no visible plaques were observed with dilution 10^{-1}; however, microscopic areas of CPE were detected with the same dilution and occasionally with dilution 10^{-2}. With Poly I:C at 10 μg/ml plus DEAE-D, the protective activity was not as effective as with higher concentrations, though it was still quite high since almost 3 logs (99.5% inhibition) in virus titer reduction was observed. With this latter concentration of the polynucleotide a reduction in the size of the plaques was also observed.

Discussion. Previous studies have shown that interferon and interferon inducers could

TABLE III. Suppression of PFU Development in OMK Cultures Preinfected with H. saimiri by Poly I:C and DEAE-D.

Poly I:C (μg/ml)	DEAE-D (μg/ml)	H. saimiri titer (PFU/0.1 ml)	Inhibition (%)
40	0	3.3×10^4	76.5
20	0	3.0×10^4	78.5
10	0	4.9×10^4	65.0
1	0	1.0×10^5	28.5
40	50	0	100.0
20	50	0	100.0
10	50	3.3×10^2	99.5
1	50	1.2×10^5	14.2
0	50	1.5×10^5	0.0
0	0 (control)	1.4×10^5	—

partially inhibit the replication of some members of the herpesvirus group, as well as to delay the development of certain virus-induced leukemias and the growth of some tumors in animals (1–9). These studies led us to search for the possibility that H. saimiri, a recently recognized oncogenic herpesvirus (10, 11) could be controlled in its replication and oncogenic activity by interferon inducers.

Most herpesvirus infections tend to develop long-term carrier states which are not necessarily eliminated by the presence of circulating antibodies. Besides, some herpesviruses have been reported to be poor producers of interferon (1, 16, 17) and also to be relatively resistant to the action of interferon (1, 18). Glasgow et al. (1) think that the capacity of some of these viruses to circumvent the host interferon response may be one of the factors related to chronic infection by these agents. However, recent reports have indicated that potent interferon inducers can be effectively used for the treatment of herpes simplex keratitis in rabbits (2, 5), as well as to reduce the mortality in mice due to encephalitis produced by intracerebral administration of the same virus (6). Based on these findings, the suggestion has been made that animal infections produced by some herpesviruses may be treated with synthetic polynucleotides (4, 6).

The present results indicate that H. saimiri, like other herpesviruses, seems to be relatively resistant to a short-term treatment of the cells with virus-induced interferon. The interferon used in these experiments only delayed the appearance of H. saimiri-produced CPE and decreased the spread of cell destruction while the same interferon diluted 1:64 produced 50% plaque reduction of VSV. The relative effectiveness with which the cells are protected against H. saimiri, seems to depend upon the length of time that interferon is in contact with the cultures. Monolayers kept in interferon medium after infection were more effectively protected.

As reported for Herpesvirus hominis (3, 5) and for a human cytomegalovirus strain (4), microgram amounts of poly I:C induced effective resistance against a direct challenge with H. saimiri in OMK cells pretreated with the synthetic polynucleotide. The protective activity was even more remarkably enhanced when Poly I:C was added together with DEAE-D into the media previously or 1 hr after the infection of the cells (Expts. 3 and 4).

The observed potentiation of the protective activity of Poly I:C by the addition of DEAE-D, even in previously infected cells, might open new possibilities to study the means to increase the resistance of susceptible nonhuman primates against the malignancy produced by H. saimiri. At this point, however, it is important to consider the possibility that H. saimiri during its replication may be actually blocking the mechanism of interferon production, the immune response or perhaps both of these. These possibilities deserve investigation.

Summary. The sensitivity of H. saimiri to virus-induced interferon and to the synthetic polynucleotide Poly I:C was determined in OMK cell cultures. These studies indicated that H. saimiri is relatively insensitive to the interferon activity in cultures pretreated for 6 hr with NDV-induced interferon. The degree of protection was improved when the cells were kept in interferon medium after the challenge with the virus. A direct pretreatment of the cells with low doses of Poly I:C induced a good protection which was greatly increased by a simultaneous addition of DEAE-D in the medium. The action of the Poly I:C/DEAE-D complex was considerably more effective when the treatment was initiated 1 hr after the inoculation of the virus. These findings suggest that the use of synthetic polynucleotides might prove to be useful for the inhibition of the malignancy produced by H. saimiri in susceptible nonhuman primates.

We are indebted to Mrs. Alice Preville for her able technical assistance and also to Mrs. Marjorie Vallee.

1. Glasgow, L. A., Hanshaw, J. B., Merigan, T. C., and Petralli, J. K., Proc. Soc. Exp. Biol. Med. 125, 843 (1967).

2. Park, J. H., and Baron, S., Science 162, 811 (1968).

3. Field, A. K., Tytell, A. A., Lampson, G. P., and Hilleman, M. R., Proc. Nat. Acad. Sci. U.S.A. 61, 340 (1968).

4. Rabson, A. S., Tyrrell, S. A., and Levy, H., Proc. Soc. Exp. Biol. Med. 131, 495 (1969).

5. Hamilton, L. C., Babcock, V. I., and Southam, C. M., Proc. Nat. Acad. Sci. U.S.A. 64, 878 (1969).

6. Catalano, L. W., Jr., and Baron, S., Proc. Soc. Exp. Biol. Med 133, 684 (1970).

7. Gresser, I., Coppey, J., and Bourali, C., J. Nat. Cancer Inst. 43, 1083 (1969).

8. Larson, V. M., Panteleakis, P. N., and Hilleman, M. R., Proc. Soc. Exp. Biol. Med. 133, 14 (1970).

9. Gelboin, H. V., and Levy, H. B., Science 167, 205 (1970).

10. Meléndez, L. V., Daniel, M. D., Hunt, R. D., Fraser, C. E. O., García, F. G., King, N. W., and Williamson, M. E., J. Nat. Cancer Inst. 44, 1175 (1970).

11. Daniel, M. D., Meléndez, L. V., Hunt, R. D., King, N. W., and Williamson, M. E., Bacteriol. Proc. 70, 165 (1970).

12. Barahona, H. H., and Hanson, R. P., Avian Dis. 12, 151 (1968).

13. Wagner, R. R., Levy, A. H., and Smith, T. J.,

in "Methods in Virology" (K. Maramorosch and H. Koprowski, eds.), Vol. 4, p. 1. Academic Press, New York (1968).

14. Dianzani, P., Cantagalli, P., Gagnoni, S., and Rita, G., Proc. Soc. Exp. Biol. Med. **128,** 703 (1968).

15. Vilcek, J., Ng, M. H., Friedman-Kien, A. E., and Krawciw, T., J. Virol. **2,** 648 (1968).

16. Vaczi, L., Horvath, E., and Hadhazy, G., Acta Microbiol. Acad. Sci. Hung. **12,** 345 (1965/66).

17. Osborn, J. E., and Medearis, D. N., Jr., Proc. Soc. Exp. Biol. Med. **121,** 819 (1965/66).

18. Cantell, K., and Tommila, F., Lancet **2,** 682 (1960).

INACTIVATION OF INFECTIOUS LARYNGOTRACHEITIS VIRUS BY DISINFECTANTS

B. W. ELLERY, B.Sc., and D. W. HOWES, M.Sc., Ph.D.

Introduction

Infectious laryngotracheitis (ILT) virus vaccine is frequently administered to chickens by either the cloacal or the ocular routes, but vaccination by incorporating virus in drinking water is an alternative method, which is simpler and more economical. Raggi and Lee (1965) and Sinkovic et al (1969) have established that this method is effective in the field. However, if vaccination is carried out using normal drinking vessels, it is possible that the vaccine virus may be inactivated by residual disinfectant remaining after the utensils have been cleaned.

Howes et al (1962) have shown that both the magnitude and frequency of protective responses which follow vaccination by the cloacal route are governed by the concentration of ILT virus in the vaccine and, in the absence of evidence to the contrary, this should be assumed to be true also for vaccines given by other routes. Therefore, where the drinking water vaccination method is used, it is important to establish that the vaccine virus will not be exposed to inactivating agents prior to its consumption.

The present study was undertaken to establish the extent to which ILT virus is inactivated by some of the more common disinfectants and the value of skim milk as a potential additive to protect against such inactivation. This readily available additive has been used to stabilise other viruses and has been shown by Jordan et al (1967) to stabilise ILT virus.

Because of the possibility of simultaneous administration of more than one medicament in drinking water, the effects of two drinking water

120

additives, an anthelmintic preparation and an anti-histomonad compound, on the infectivity of ILT virus were also examined.

Materials and Methods

Virus

A crude suspension of the SA_2 strain (vaccine strain) of ILT virus grown in embryonic chicken kidney (CEK) cells was used. Infected monolayers were harvested and, after centrifugation at 150 x g, cells were resuspended in phosphate buffered saline pH 6.6 (PBS 6.6) containing penicillin, streptomycin and amphotericin B (100 iu/ml, 100 μg/ml and 100 μg/ml respectively). Cells in the suspension were then disrupted by ultrasonic vibration, and the debris was removed by centrifugation at 1700 x g.

Disinfectants

Disinfectants tested were of two basic types:—
(1) Quaternary ammonium chlorides of the benzyl-alkyl-ammonium chloride type consisting of complex mixtures of n-alkyldimethylbenzylammonium (benzalkonium) chlorides with the alkyl groups ranging from C_8 (caprylyl) to C_{16} (palmityl). The distribution of the various components within a preparation may vary widely from one product to another (Reubner *et al* 1970). Five different preparations of this type were examined and for identification purposes they have been designated 1 to 5.*

(2) Substituted xylene† consisting ot 2-4-dichloro-meta-xylenol plus a soap.

Medicaments

The drinking water anthelmintic additive for treatment of round worms was piperazine and the anti-histomonad‡ contained the active ingredient 2-acetylamino-5-nitrothiazole.

Skim Milk

Powdered skim milk was reconstituted in PBS 6.6 before use.

Water

In the experiment testing the effect of the agents in water, Melbourne metropolitan tap water was used.

---

*The use of particular brand-name products is not to be construed as either a recommendation or a reprobation. Results suggest that products which have a similar content of active ingredient will have quantitatively similar effects on the infectivity of ILT virus. Products examined were:—
1. Germtox 10% (Croda Federal Chemicals Ltd., Richmond North, Victoria).
2. Sanicide (Leonard Chemical Products Pty. Ltd., Notting Hill, Victoria).
3. Water-san (Clarke King & Co. Pty. Ltd., Melbourne, Victoria).
4. Poultone 10% (Swan Chemical Industries, Moorabbin, Victoria).
5. Zephiran (Bayer Pharma Pty. Ltd., Ermington, New South Wales).

†Germ-i-san (Clarke King & Co., Pty. Ltd., Melbourne Victoria).

‡Piperazine Solution and Nitrazole (Biological Institute of Australasia Pty. Ltd., Sydney, NSW). Piperazine Solution contains 17% w/v of piperazine as piperazine chloride.

121

TABLE 1

Effect of Medicaments on Infectivity of ILT Virus

Diluent	Preparation	Concentration of Active Ingredient In Reaction Mixture* (%)	Experiment 1		Experiment 2	
			Plaques Counted	Survival of Virus (%)	Plaques Counted	Survival of Virus (%)
PBS 6.6†	Nil	—	37	100	143	100
	Piperazine	0.32	35	97	154	107
	2-acetylamino-5-nitrothiazole	0.022	37	100	177	123
Water	Nil	—	ND	ND	138	96
	Piperazine	0.32	ND	ND	158	110
	2-acetylamino-5-nitrothiazole	0.022	ND	ND	161	112

*Reaction mixture contained equal amounts of virus suspension and the medication under test. After incubation for 30 minutes at room temperature the mixture was further diluted and residual virus was assayed.
†Phosphate buffered saline pH 6.6.

122

Titration of Virus

To study the virus-inactivating capacities of the preparations, various dilutions of each in either PBS 6.6 or tap water were mixed with an equal volume of ILT virus suspension, and after 30 minutes at room temperature (approximately 25°C) the mixture was diluted at least 10^{-3} in PBS 6.6. Residual virus was assayed by counting plaques produced in monolayer cultures of CEK cells with minor modifications to the method described by Howes *et al* (1962).

When the effect of skim milk was examined, it was added to the virus suspension to a concentration of 2% before disinfectant was added.

Results

Effect of Medicaments on Virus Infectivity

As shown in Table 1, piperazine and 2-acetylamino-5-nitrothiazole had no detectable effect on the infectivity of ILT virus, when used at or below, the concentration recommended by the manufacturer. The deviations from 100% survival are not significant. Both products behave similarly in PBS 6.6 and tap water.

The manufacturer recommends that, for medicinal use for young birds the anthelmintic solution be diluted 1/53, which gives a 0.32% (w/v) solution of piperazine. The recommended dilution of the antihistomonad for medicinal use is 1/640, which yields a 0.025% (w/v) solution of 2-acetylamino-5-nitrothiazole.

Effect of Disinfectants on the Infectivity of ILT Virus

When ILT virus was incubated with any of the disinfectants examined, less than 0.13% survived when the disinfectant concentration was that recommended by the manufacturer for disinfecting purposes (Table 2).

However, as is shown in the typical examples of Figures 1 and 2 (broken lines), when the disinfectants were further diluted to one hundredth of the recommended concentration none caused any detectable virus inactivation. All of the products containing benzyl-alkyl-ammonium chlorides behaved similarly to the example shown in Figure 1, which shows that ILT virus was not detectably inactivated within 30 minutes at room temperature when the concentration of quaternary ammonium chlorides was less than 0.001%. Figure 2 indicates that no inactivation of ILT virus could be detected when 0.00015% or less of 2,4-dichloro-meta-xylenol was present. The disinfectants behaved similarly in both PBS 6.6 and tap water.

Protective Effect of Skim Milk

Skim milk partially protected ILT virus against

123

TABLE 2

Survival of ILT Virus after Incubation with Disinfectants at Concentrations Recommended by Manufacturers for Disinfecting

Type of Product	Product identification number	Reciprocal of Final Dilution of Product in Reaction Mixture*	Active Ingredient in Reaction Mixture (%)†	Survival of ILT Virus			
				Experiment 1		Experiment 2	
				Plaques	% of control count	Plaques	% of control count
Control	—	—	—	37	100	162	100
Benzalkonium chloride	1	560	0.02	0	< 0.28	0	< 0.13
	2	80	0.15	0	< 0.28	0	< 0.13
	3	160	0.06	0	< 0.54	0	< 0.13
	4	80	0.13	0	< 0.28	0	< 0.13
	5	1000	0.01	0	< 0.28	0	< 0.13
2,4-dichloro-meta-xylenol	6	80	0.02	2	5.4	0	< 0.13

*Reaction mixture contained mixture of virus and product under test. This was allowed to react for 30 minutes at room temperature and, after further dilution, residual virus was assayed.
†Figures based on content of either quaternary ammonium chloride or substituted xylenol in product.

124

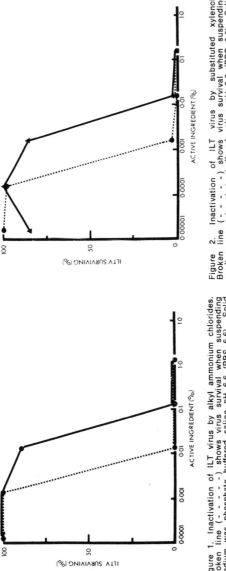

Figure 1. Inactivation of ILT virus by alkyl ammonium chlorides. Broken line (- - - -) shows virus survival when suspending medium was phosphate buffered saline pH 6.6 (PBS 6.6). Solid line (————) shows survival in presence of 1% skim milk in PBS 6.6.

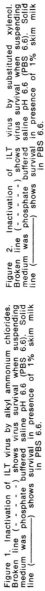

Figure 2. Inactivation of ILT virus by substituted xylenol. Broken line (- - - -) shows virus survival when suspending medium was phosphate buffered saline pH 6.6 (PBS 6.6). Solid line (————) shows survival in presence of 1% skim milk in PBS 6.6.

125

inactivation by both types of disinfectants examined. Figures 1 and 2 show that the amount of active ingredient needed to reduce the surviving fraction of ILT virus to less than 10% was approximately ten times larger when 1% skim milk was present (solid lines) than when the virus was suspended in PBS 6.6 only (broken lines).

Discussion

If vaccination against ILT by drinking water is to be successful the vaccine virus should remain viable until all the medicated water has been consumed. This study has shown that ILT virus is readily inactivated by commonly used disinfectants of both the benzyl-alkyl-ammonium chloride and substituted xylenol types at the concentrations recommended by manufacturers for general disinfection. Consequently ILT virus vaccine should not be administered in drinking water containing products designed to prevent bacterial and fungal contamination of the water, and it is prudent to rinse residual disinfectant from washed drinking vessels before vaccine is added to the drinking water.

Under these conditions there seems to be little likelihood that the vaccine virus will be inactivated by disinfectant prior to its consumption, but a greater safety margin is afforded by the inclusion of 1% skim milk in the water to which ILT virus vaccine is added. In 1% skim milk, ten times as much disinfectant is needed to inactivate ILT virus as in buffer alone and, even where drinking vessels are not rinsed, it is unlikely that the vaccine virus would be substantially inactivated by residual disinfectants if skim milk is included.

The medicaments examined do not inactivate ILT virus under the conditions used but administration of combinations of medicaments and vaccines in drinking water should be approached with caution until more is known of the interactions between various additives.

Summary

ᵛThe effect of several commercial disinfectants on the infectivity of infectious laryngotracheitis virus was studied. Benzalkonium chlorides did not cause any detectable inactivation of the virus when their concentration was less than 0.001%, but at concentrations greater than 0.01% no surviving virus was detected.

At 0.00015% 2,4-dichloro-meta-xylenol did

126

not detectably inactivate virus, while no virus survived in the presence of 0.01% of the compound.

In the presence of 1% skim milk, ten times as much disinfectant was needed to inactivate the same amount of virus.

An anthelmintic and an anti-histomonad had no detectable effect on virus infectivity at concentrations of 0.32% and 0.025% respectively.

The significance of the findings in relation to vaccination of poultry against infectious laryngotracheitis via drinking water is discussed.

Acknowledgments
The technical assistance of Miss M. Imberg, Miss L. Barnes, Mrs. M. Ford, and Mr. W. Zarifeh is gratefully acknowledged.

References
Howes, D. W., Tannock, G. A., and Sinkovic, B. (1962)—*Proc. XIIth Worlds Poultry Congress,* Sydney, p. 244.
Jordan, F. T. W., Evanson, H. M., Bennett, J. M. (1967)—*Zbl. Vet. Med. B,* **14:** 135.
Raggi, L. C., and Lee, G. G. (1965)—*Poultry Sci.* **44:** 509.
Reubner, H. W., Rude, T. A., and Jorgenson, I. A. (1970)—*Avian Dis.,* **14:** 211.
Sinkovic, B., Littlejohns, I. R., Howes, D. W., and Tannock, G. A. (1969)—*Proc. Aust. Poultry Sci. Conv.,* Surfers Paradise, p. 347.
Sinkovic, B., Watson, A. R. A., Littlejohns, I. R., Jackson, C. A. W., Howes, D. W., and White, N. J. (1969)—*Proc. Aust. Poultry Sci. Conv.,* Surfers Paradise, p. 363.

Host-cell reactivation in mammalian cells
III. Effect of caffeine on herpes virus survival

C. DAVID LYTLE

Survival curves of u.v.-irradiated herpes virus have been determined in the presence of different caffeine concentrations. At low concentrations (which do not greatly reduce virus plaque-forming ability), the first component of the survival curves was only slightly affected, whereas the slope of the second component was increased. At higher concentrations, the slope of the first component increased and the fraction of infected cells expressing the second component decreased. Since repair replication in u.v.-irradiated cells is not reduced by caffeine, the caffeine sensitivity of irradiated herpes virus suggests a second recovery mechanism for the virus. The caffeine sensitivity decreased at the time viral DNA synthesis normally commences, implying a correlation of caffeine-sensitive u.v. recovery with viral DNA synthesis.

1. Introduction

For a virus particle harbouring damage from ultra-violet irradiation, one of the most important factors controlling its survival is the degree to which the u.v. lesions will be repaired. Host-cell reactivation (HCR) plays a major role in the survival of u.v.-irradiated SV_{40} (Aaronson and Lytle 1970) and herpes simplex virus (Lytle 1971 b, Lytle, Aaronson and Harvey 1972).

The relation of the cellular repair mechanisms to this HCR is not completely known. Repair replication apparently accounts for at least part (Aaronson and Lytle 1970, Lytle et al. 1972). However, since caffeine lowers the survival of u.v.-irradiated herpes virus (Lytle 1970, 1971 a) and since caffeine does not affect cellular repair replication (Cleaver 1969), it seems likely that another repair mechanism may be involved. Defective mutants for such a repair capacity have not been characterized, so a direct test of this repair mechanism cannot be made. The caffeine sensitivity of virus survival, however, permits an indirect approach to investigate the possibility of another recovery mechanism being active in HCR. This paper reports the study of the effect of caffeine on irradiated virus survival. The results demonstrate that caffeine sensitivity exists for both components of the survival curve and coincides approximately with the beginning of viral DNA synthesis.

2. Materials and methods

2.1. *Virus and cells*

Herpes simplex virus (MP strain) was used in these studies. The virus assay procedure has been described (Lytle 1971 b).

CV-1 (African green monkey kidney) cells and human skin fibroblasts (developed from a skin biopsy from a 29-year-old female) were used. CV-1

128

was cultured in NCTC 109 medium, and the human cells in Eagle's MEM. In virus assays newly confluent cell monlayers in T–30 disposable plastic flasks (Falcon) were used, unless otherwise noted. The caffeine (Calbiochem, Los Angeles, California, USP grade) stock solution (2 per cent) was made in distilled water and autoclaved. This was later diluted into tissue culture media for experiments.

Caffeine in the tissue culture medium decreased plaque formation by unirradiated virus. Figure 1 shows relative plaque-forming ability at different caffeine concentrations. The plaquing efficiency decreases to 50 per cent at about 7 mM in CV–1 cells and at about 4 mM in human skin fibroblasts.

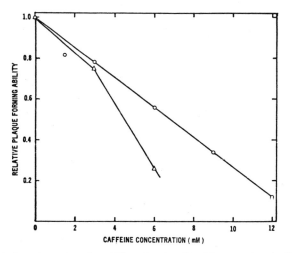

Figure 1. Relative plaque forming ability of unirradiated herpes virus in CV–1 (o) cells and human skin fibroblast (Δ) cells at different caffeine concentrations.

2.2. *Irradiation*

A germicidal u.v. lamp (254 nm) was used to irradiate virus suspensions. The procedure has been previously described (Lytle 1971 b).

3. Results
3.1. *Effect of different caffeine concentrations on typical herpes virus survival curves*

To characterize the caffeine inhibition of HCR, survival curves were obtained in CV–1 cells for several different caffeine concentrations (figure 2). Medium containing the caffeine was added to infected assay cultures at the end of the 1½ hour virus adsorption period. Changes in the first component of these two component curves were difficult to ascertain from figure 2. However, the second component showed two major changes: the slope increased at low caffeine concentrations, but was nearer the usual value at higher concentrations; the intercept extrapolated to zero dose decreased only at high caffeine concentrations. The differences in responses to high and low caffeine concentrations suggest that there was more than one effect elicited by the presence of caffeine.

129

The quantitative aspects of the different survival curves are summarized in the table. For a given component, the U.V. dose (e^{-1} dose) necessary to give an average of one lethal hit per virus is measured as that dose which gives a survival of 37 per cent of that at zero dose.

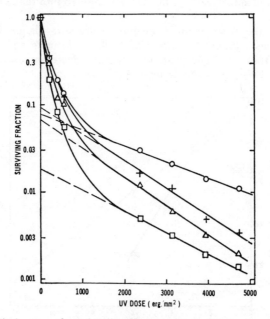

Figure 2. Survival curves of U.V.-irradiated herpes virus in CV–1 cells at different caffeine concentrations: ○—no caffeine; +—3 mM; △—6 mM; □—9 mM.

The caffeine effect on the first component was examined by first subtracting the second component from the total survival curve. The resultant curves are shown in figure 3. These data show that caffeine lowered the survival slightly. Since the curves were not straight lines, as is usually found when the first components are resolved (Lytle 1971 b), the slopes at low U.V. doses were used to calculate the e^{-1} doses.

Caffeine concentration	CV–1 component (erg/mm²)		Human skin fibroblast (erg/mm²)
	I	II	
0	170	2400	210
3 mM	170	1400	200
6 mM	150	1350	130
9 mM	120	1800	—

Dose for an average of one lethal hit (e^{-1} dose) to U.V.-irradiated herpes virus at different caffeine concentrations.

R.B.   M

130

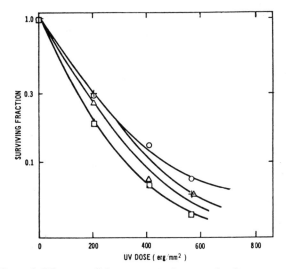

Figure 3. Effect of different caffeine concentrations on the first component of herpes virus survival curves in CV–1 cells: O—no caffeine; + —3 mM; Δ—6 mM; □—9 mM.

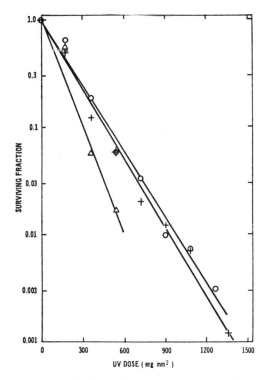

Figure 4. Survival curves of u.v.-irradiated herpes virus on human skin fibroblasts (confluent monolayers for 10 days before infection) at different caffeine concentrations; O—no caffeine; + —3 mM; Δ—6 mM.

131

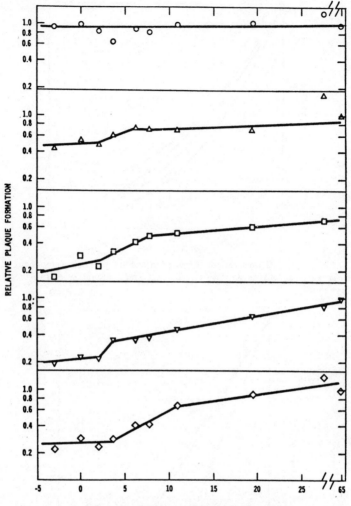

RELATIVE PLAQUE FORMATION

TIME AFTER INFECTION OF CAFFEINE ADDITION (HOURS)

Figure 5. Time dependence of caffeine inhibition of plaque formation by control and irradiated herpes virus in CV–1 cells. Plaque formation relative to that obtained in the absence of caffeine is represented for each u.v. dose. Caffeine (3 mM) was added at the times indicated relative to the end of the virus adsorption period (0 hours). u.v. dose to the virus: ○—control; △—1750 erg/mm²; □—2625 erg/mm²; ▽—3500 erg/mm²; ◇—4375 erg/mm².

To look at a first component more directly, survival curves which normally have only one component were used in similar caffeine concentration experiments. Some cell-types give single-component survival curves if they have been kept confluent for some time before use in assay of u.v.-irradiated herpes virus (Lytle 1971 a). Human skin fibroblasts that had been confluent for ten days were used, and the survival curves at different caffeine concentrations are presented in figure 4. As with the first component in CV–1 cells, 3 mM caffeine had little effect, whereas 6 mM produced a distinctly greater slope. The e^{-1} doses are presented in the table.

3.2. Time of recovery

The above data demonstrate that caffeine reduced the survival of irradiated virus. Therefore the addition of caffeine at a time before the recovery mechanism can act should inhibit its expression, whereas addition after the recovery has occurred should not have this effect. An experiment testing this principle was conducted with 3 mM caffeine, a concentration that had only a small effect on control virus plaque formation (figure 1) or cell growth (unpublished observation). The experimental procedure was as follows: confluent cells were infected, incubated in normal medium at 37°c, and at different times medium containing 3 mM caffeine was substituted.

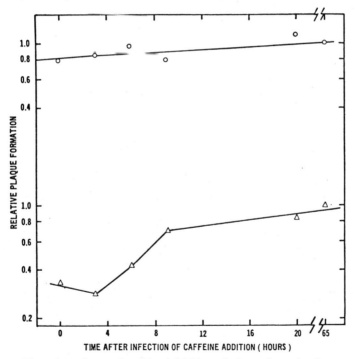

Figure 6. Time dependence of caffeine inhibition of plaque formation by control and irradiated herpes virus in human skin fibroblasts. Plaque formation relative to that obtained in the absence of caffeine is represented for each u.v. dose. Caffeine (3 mM) was added at the times indicated relative to the end of the virus adsorption period (0 hours). u.v. dose to virus: ○—control; △—720 erg/mm².

133

Data obtained in CV–1 cells for irradiated and control viruses (the doses used place survival in the second component of the survival curve) are shown in figure 5; for the human skin fibroblasts (single-component survival only) in figure 6. These data show that caffeine added before about 4 hours after infection inhibited plaque formation for irradiated virus which was no longer caffeine-sensitive after about 10 hours. Control virus was slightly caffeine-sensitive, although the step between 4 and 10 hours after infection occurred only for irradiated virus.

4. Discussion

The data presented here demonstrated a decrease in survival for u.v.-irradiated herpes virus in monkey and human cells when caffeine was present. Since herpes virus is apparently three times more sensitive to u.v. when assayed in xeroderma pigmentosum cells than in normal human cells for both components of the survival curves (Lytle et al. 1972), host-cell reactivation by the cellular repair replication mechanism probably accounts for about 70 per cent of the recovery of irradiated virus in each component. However, since repair replication in human cells (HeLa) is not inhibited by 1 mM or 10 mM caffeine (Cleaver 1969), the caffeine sensitivity of u.v.-irradiated herpes virus survival suggests the presence of a second recovery mechanism in each component.

At caffeine concentrations which decreased virus plaque-forming ability less than 50 per cent (i.e. below 7 mM for CV–1 and below 4 mM for human skin), there was apparently only a small effect on the slopes of the first components. At these concentrations, there was a definite increase in slope of the second component in monkey kidney cells. A similar change at 2·5 mM caffeine in the second component of the survival curve for u.v.-irradiated pseudo-rabies virus has been reported (Závadová and Závada 1968). At caffeine concentrations which greatly affected virus plaque-forming ability, the first component slopes increased. This differential effect on the two components suggests that possibly the mechanisms producing the two components are different. The fact that the fraction of infected cells expressing the second component decreased at high caffeine concentrations may be related to reduced growth of the host cells (Lytle 1970).

There is evidence that a caffeine-sensitive recovery mechanism from u.v. damage exists in mammalian cells (Rauth 1967, Domon and Rauth 1969). Domon and Rauth (1969) have shown that the colony-forming ability of u.v.-irradiated mouse L cells was reduced if 2 mM caffeine were present during the first DNA synthesis phase after irradiation. This correlation of caffeine-sensitive u.v. recovery and DNA synthesis in the cell may also be applicable to the virus situation. DNA synthesis of unirradiated herpes virus begins about 4 hours after infection in human cells (HEp-2) (Roizman, Aurelian and Roane 1963) and in monkey kidney cells (BSC-1) (Olshevsky, Levitt and Becker 1967). Thus the time of caffeine inhibition of plaque formation for irradiated virus coincides with the time of initiation of viral DNA synthesis. Therefore a mechanism may be functioning for irradiated virus which is similar to that for irradiated cells. The relation of this recovery process to currently known repair or photoproduct bypass mechanisms is not understood (Cleaver and Thomas 1969, Humphrey 1971).

134

It is only by analogy with the cellular caffeine-sensitive recovery that this viral recovery might be considered as HCR. There is no evidence that this 'reactivation' is controlled by the host cell. The caffeine-sensitive process may be a manifestation of viral-controlled synthesis of irradiated DNA (Cleaver and Thomas 1969).

ACKNOWLEDGMENTS

I gratefully acknowledge the generous gift of the human skin fibroblast culture from Dr. E. J. Pollock. I also wish to thank Mrs. S. Benane for excellent technical assistance. I thank Drs. L. E. Bockstahler and C. F. Blackman for critical review of the manuscript.

Des courbes de survie de virus herpétiques, irradiés aux u.v., ont été déterminées, en présence de caféine à différentes concentrations. A basses concentrations (ne réduisant pas de façon significative la capacité des virus à former des plaques), la première composante des courbes de survie n'était que légèrement modifiée, tandis que la pente de la deuxième composante était augmentée. A des concentrations plus élevées, la pente de la première composante était accrue, et la proportion de cellules infectées exprimant la seconde composante diminuait. Etant donné que la caféine ne réduit pas la réplication de réparation dans les cellules irradiés par les u.v., la sensibilité à la caféine des virus herpétiques irradiés, suggère l'existence d'un second mécanisme de réparation pour ces virus. La sensibilité à la caféine diminuait au même moment où la synthèse d'ADN viral commençait dans les cellules en l'absence de caféine, impliquant une corrélation entre la synthèse d'ADN viral et la composante de la réparation des lésions induits par les u.v. et sensible à la caféine.

Unter Gegenwart verschiedener Koffeinkonzentrationen wurden Überlebenskurven von u.v.-bestrahltem Herpes-Virus bestimmt. Bei niedrigen Konzentrationen (welche geringen reduzierenden Einfluss auf das Plaque-bildungsvermögen haben) war die erste Komponente der Überlebenskurve nur wenig beeinflusst, während der Verlauf der zweiten Komponente anstieg. Bei höheren Konzentrationen stieg der Verlauf der ersten Komponente an, während der Fraktion infizierter Zellen (die zweite Komponente darstellend) abnahm. Weil die Reparaturreplikation in u.v.-bestrahlten Zellen bei Anwesenheit von Koffein nicht reduziert ist, lässt die Koffeinempfindlichkeit von bestrahlten Herpes Virus einen zweiten Wiederherstellungsmechanismus vermuten. Die Koffeinsensitivität liess nach mit dem normalen Beginn der Virus DNS-synthese, was eine Korrelation zwischen koffeinsensitiver u.v.-Bestrahlungsreparatur und Virus DNS-Synthese vermuten lässt.

REFERENCES

AARONSON, S. A., and LYTLE, C. D., 1970, Nature, Lond., 228, 359.
CLEAVER, J. E., 1969, Radiat. Res., 37, 334.
CLEAVER, J. E., and THOMAS, G. H., 1969, Biochem. biophys. Res. Commun., 36, 203.
DOMON, M., and RAUTH, A. M., 1969, Radiat. Res., 40, 414.
HUMPHREY, R. M., 1971, Nineteenth Annual Meeting of the Radiation Research Society, Boston, Massachusetts, 9–13 May.
LYTLE, C. D., 1970, NASA Symposium on Extreme Environments, Moffett Field, California, 24–26 June; 1971 a, Nineteenth Annual Meeting of the Radiation Research Society, Boston, Massachusetts, 9–13 May; 1971 b, Int. J. Radiat. Biol., 19, 329.
LYTLE, C. D., AARONSON, S. A., and HARVEY, E., 1972, Int. J. Radiat. Biol., 22, 159.
OLSHEVSKY, U., LEVITT, J., and BECKER, Y., 1967, Virology, 33, 323.
RAUTH, A. M., 1967, Radiat. Res., 31, 121.
ROIZMAN, B., AURELIAN, L., and ROANE, P. R., Jr., 1963, Virology, 21, 482.
ZÁVADOVÁ, Z., and ZÁVADA, J., 1968, Acta virol., Prague, 12, 507.

Herpes simplex:
Diagnosis and management

A. P. ULBRICH, D.O., FAOCD

A layman often can diagnose correctly a case
of ordinary herpes simplex, primarily because
of the accustomed location of the lesions in
the perioral area, and secondly because of the
characteristic repetition of herpetic lesions at
the original point of infection during subsequent episodes of the disease. In fact, if the
lesions do not follow this pattern, the diagnosis
should be in doubt until confirmed by laboratory tests. Primary herpes simplex would,
of course, be an exception.

Dermatologists generally are aware of the
unusual manifestations of skin disease and
know that herpes simplex lesions are not con-
fined to the oral area.[1] However, many doctors
assume as does the layman that it is an oral
problem only. Herpetic lesions can occur on
other parts of the body. (The genital area is
the second most affected area.) Recent pathologic studies are leading to a better understanding of herpes simplex, as well as its relationship to other diseases.

The morphologic structure of herpetic lesions is the same; no matter where the vesicles
occur on the body, they are seen as multi-

locular groups of superficial vesicles. Bullae occur only under extenuating circumstances. Two types of herpes simplex can be identified, however. Type I herpes simplex develops above the clavicle; Type II occurs in the genital area. Herpetic lesions on the torso can be either, and both types may be present at the same time.

In a tissue culture, Type I herpesvirus hominis is shown to produce smaller pocks than Type II.[2] A Type I culture also shows a preference for the ectoderm; there is little subectodermal involvement. Type II, on the other hand, involves ectodermal, mesodermal, and endodermal change, as seen in tissue cultures. These types can be differentiated in a special neutralization kinetic procedure and through a fluorescent technique.[2]

Differentiating herpes simplex as to type is important in two respects. First, although still in the investigative stage, a vaccine has been prepared from Type I. It is only effective, however, in decreasing the incidence of Type I lesions and is not currently available. Second, apparently there is some relationship between Type II herpes simplex and carcinoma of the cervix. The titer ratio to herpes simplex is higher in carcinomas of the cervix, both in carcinomas in situ and in massive carcinomas. One report of histologically confirmed cases showed high titers in all cases.[3]

The herpes virus is made up of DNA nucleic acids. One cell is 100-200 mμ in diameter with 162 capsomeres projecting from its capsular membrane. The growth of herpes simplex disease follows the basic cycle of any virus attack on mammals. According to Bell,[4] the first stage is adsorption, or the attachment of the virus to the cell wall, which is followed by penetration, when the virus passes through the cell wall and enters the cytoplasm. The eclipse stage is difficult to comprehend, as the virus in this stage cannot be detected in the cell. It is thought, however, that during this time the virus assumes command of the

137

host cell's metabolism and reorganizes the cell system for reproduction of the virus. Replication follows with the manufacture of separate component parts of the virus. In herpes simplex replication occurs in the nucleus rather than in the cytoplasm. Maturation is the fitting together of the component parts and the formation of the capsule (probably the antigenic portion). The final phase, release, occurs when the infected cell bursts, releasing the complete virus. Release can also be a gradual extrusion of virus cells from dead or dying host cells.

The disease herpes simplex is the result of an episode of growth of herpesvirus hominis. As the clinical manifestation may be a localized allergic reaction to the virus, rather than a reaction to circulating antibodies, use of the word "result" is preferable to infection or reinfection. An episode of herpes simplex does not increase the titer of circulating antibodies; the number remains constant. Apparently the antibody cannot penetrate the wall of the invaded cell, and since the virus is within the nucleus of its host, the antibody cannot attack the virus. Although there are two types of herpes simplex, there is only one type of antibody to herpesvirus hominis. Antibodies taken from individuals with herpes simplex react to both Type I and Type II viruses.

Signs of the first episode of herpes simplex are extremely variable.[4] It is estimated that clinical symptoms are evident in only ten percent of the cases. The most common manifestations are upper respiratory infections or gingivostomatitis, but primary disease can also be seen as regional vesiculation. The incubation period of herpes simplex is from two to 12 days. Herpes simplex is considered an occupational hazard to dentists and anesthetists because minor lacerations on fingers can become avenues for a primary virus.[5]

When steroids are applied topically to active herpes simplex, they increase the carbohydrate metabolism of the viral particle while inhibiting the cytopathologic effect of the virus. The result is an increase in the number and spread of virus.[4] Similar results are seen in cases of herpes simplex and verruca when immunosuppressive drugs are administered.[6] (Herpes zoster can also occur in patients who are taking immunosuppressive drugs.) A recent publication reports a case of generalized herpes simplex occurring in a patient who was receiving heavy doses of a steroid for pemphigus.[7] The patient's axillae and groin were particularly affected, although the disease did not persist longer than its usual 14-day course.

Patients who state that they have chronic shingles actually suffer from aberrant herpes simplex. Only rarely does herpes zoster recur. When it does, the affected area is seldom the original site of infection, as is characteristic of herpes simplex.[8] In cases of recurring zoster, a malignancy such as lymphoma or Hodgkins disease should be suspected. Viral cultures have also proved the possibility of the existence of herpes simplex and herpes zoster in a patient at the same time; the simplex outbreak occurs in the usual location, the varicella in another area.[9]

1. Ulbrich, A.P., and Schweig, E.: Herpes simplex. JAOA 62:720-4, Apr 63

2. Kopf, A.W., and Andrade, R.: Yearbook of dermatology, 1969. Yearbook Medical Publishers, Chicago

3. Royston, L., et al.: Genital herpes virus findings in relation to cervical neoplasia. J Reprod Med 4:109-13, Apr 70

4. Bell, T.M.: An introduction to general virology. J.B. Lippincott Co., Philadelphia, 1965

5. Hambrick, G.W., Jr., Cox, R.P., and Senior, J.R.: Primary herpes simplex infection of fingers of medical personnel. Arch Derm, Chicago 85:583-9, May 62

6. Medical World News. Outlook section. 11:13, 28 Aug 70

7. Indgin, S.N., Katz, S.I., and Connor, J.D.: Pemphigus and herpes simplex. Antibody response to corticosteroids in a patient. Arch Derm (Chicago) 102:333-6, Sep 70

8. Crittenden, F.M., and Sire, D.J.: Recurrent Zoster. Cutis 6:877-80, Aug 70

9. Kahn, G.: Zoster and herpes simplex. Simultaneous occurrence in same patient. Arch Derm (Chicago) 95:298, Mar 67

Templeton, A.C.: Generalized herpes simplex in malnourished children. J Clin Path 23:24-30, Feb 70

Differential Effect of 7,12-Dimethylbenz[a]anthracene on Infectivity of Herpes Simplex Virus Type 2[1]

JOHN J. DOCHERTY, ROBERT J. GOLDBERG, AND FRED RAPP

Herpes simplex virus (HSV) has been subdivided into 2 groups based on the area from which the viruses were isolated; either oral or genital. Although the basis for grouping oral isolates as type 1 and genital isolates as type 2 is serological (1, 2), the 2 types differ in other biological characteristics. These differences include pock formation on the chorioallantoic membrane of embryonated hen eggs, plaque formation in chick embryo cell cultures and neurovirulence in mice (3, 4).

A variety of studies have shown an association of herpesviruses with numerous types of cancer (5–11), and epidemiological studies have suggested a link of HSV-type 2 to human cervical carcinoma (12). In addition, it is known that certain chemicals can act as carcinogenic agents. One of the most potent chemical compounds with this property is 7,12-dimethylbenz[a]anthracene (DMBA).

In our studies we have noted that DMBA, a carcinogenic polycyclic aromatic hydrocarbon, has a preferential effect on HSV-type 2 rather than on HSV-type 1. Our results have shown HSV-type 2 is more sensitive to DMBA than type 1 as measured by inactivation of infectivity.

Materials and Methods. Primary rabbit kidney (RK) cultures. Monolayer cultures were grown in 1-oz prescription bottles and

[1] This study was conducted under Contract No. 70-2024 within the Special Virus-Cancer Program of the National Cancer Institute, NIH, PHS.

60×15-mm plastic petri dishes as previously described (13). The medium used for cell cultivation consisted of 10% bovine serum in Eagle's basal medium with 0.075% $NaHCO_3$ (closed cultures) or 0.23% $NaHCO_3$ (open cultures). Each ml of the medium was additionally supplemented with 100 units of penicillin, 100 μg of streptomycin, 1 μg of Fungizone, and 10 units of Mycostatin.

Virus. All herpes simplex virus (HSV) strains used in this study were obtained from Dr. William Rawls, Baylor College of Medicine, Houston, Texas. Virus stocks were prepared in primary RK cells in 8-oz bottles. Infected cultures were harvested following incubation for 2 to 3 days at $37°$ at which time approximately 75% of the cells exhibited cytopathic changes. The infected cultures were ruptured by 2 cycles of alternate freezing and thawing, clarified by centrifugation at 1500 rpm for 10 min, and the supernatant fluid was collected, quick-frozen, and stored at $-65°$ until used.

Plaque assay. HSV was titrated by a modification of the plaque assay technique in RK cells under a methylcellulose overlay as previously described (13). Virus samples were diluted in 0.025 M tris(hydroxymethyl) aminoethane (Tris) saline (pH 7.4) containing 3% bovine serum and antibiotics. The virus, in 0.1-ml amounts, was inoculated into each of 2 primary RK cell cultures in 60-mm plastic dishes and adsorbed for 1 hr at room temperature with intermittent manual rotation. Each plate was then overlayed with 5 ml of Eagle's basal medium supplemented with 0.5% methylcellulose, 5% bovine serum, antibiotics and 0.23% $NaHCO_3$. Following 4 days of incubation at $37°$ in an atmosphere of 5% CO_2, the cultures were stained with a 1:7500 solution of neutral red in Tris saline. The plaques were counted 1 hr after the addition of the dye.

Virus growth studies. Primary RK cultures, grown in 1-oz prescription bottles, were drained and inoculated with 0.1-ml volumes of HSV containing 10^6 plaque-forming units (PFU). The virus was allowed to adsorb for

1 hr at room temperature with frequent rotation to insure uniform distribution of the virus inoculum. The cultures were then washed 3 times with Eagle's basal medium containing 10% fetal calf serum, antibiotics, and 0.075% $NaHCO_3$ to remove unattached virus, and overlayed with 5 ml of the same nutrient medium. Polycyclic aromatic hydrocarbons were added to the overlay medium as indicated. The bottles were incubated at 37° and sampled for production of virus at various intervals after infection. Extracellular virus was obtained by harvesting the supernatant fluids from infected cultures and rinsing the monolayers 2 times with nutrient medium. The fluids from each culture were pooled and clarified by centrifugation at 1500 rpm for 10 min at room temperature. Cell-associated virus was obtained by adding 5 ml of nutrient medium to the washed cell sheets and freezing and thawing the cultures 2 times to release intracellular virus.

Chemicals. DMBA was purchased from Eastman Organic Chemicals, Rochester, New York. Anthracene (Ant) was obtained from K & K Laboratories, Inc., Plainview, New York. Dimethylsulfoxide (DMSO) was purchased from Matheson Coleman and Bell, Norwood, Ohio. Stock solutions of DMBA or Ant were prepared with DMSO as solvent. Further dilutions of these compounds were made in Tris buffer or Eagle's nutrient medium where indicated to produce a colloidal solution.

Results. Infection of RK cells in the presence of DMBA. Initial studies were performed to study the effect of this chemcial carcinogen on the growth of a type 2 HSV. Primary RK cells, in 1-oz bottles, were infected with the 316D strain of HSV-type 2 as indicated in Materials and Methods. Infected cultures were incubated in the presence or absence of DMBA or as control, the non-carcinogenic Ant, at a final concentration of 10 μg/ml. Additional controls included infected cultures incubated in the presence of a concentration of DMSO equivalent to that used as solvent for DMBA or Ant.

TABLE I. The Effect of Noncarcinogenic and Carcinogenic Polycyclic Aromatic Hydrocarbons on Intracellular and Extracellular HSV-type 2.

| Treatment | Titer of herpes simplex virus (PFU/ml) ; time in hr | | |
	0	24	48
Extracellular virus			
None	8.5×10^2	1.3×10^5	1.8×10^5
DMBA[a]	2.5×10^1	$<10^1$	5.0×10^1
Ant[a]	4.7×10^2	6.2×10^4	2.1×10^5
DMSO[b]	7.8×10^2	5.5×10^4	2.9×10^5
Cell-associated virus			
None	2.3×10^3	1.4×10^6	1.2×10^6
DMBA	4.6×10^2	1.3×10^4	1.0×10^2
Ant	1.7×10^3	5.0×10^5	5.3×10^5
DMSO	2.4×10^3	1.9×10^6	8.0×10^5

[a] After virus adsorption the chemicals were added at a concentration of 10 μg/ml of growth medium.

[b] Dimethylsulfoxide was used as the diluent for the chemicals.

The results of this experiment are presented in Table I. It is evident that comparable virus titers were obtained in untreated and in Ant- or DMSO-treated RK cultures. The data also show that extracellular and cell-associated HSV yields were significantly reduced in infected RK cultures incubated in the presence of DMBA. The appearance of infectious extracellular virus was virtually eliminated in DMBA-treated cultures while the limited titers of cell-associated virus measured in these cultures at 24 hr decreased in the presence of this compound.

Effect of DMBA on HSV infectivity. The preceeding results suggested that the decreased HSV yields obtained in DMBA-treated cultures may have resulted from the direct inactivation of the infectivity of this virus by the chemical. This hypothesis was tested by measuring the effect of DMBA, Ant, and DMSO on the infectivity of HSV at 37°. Virus dilutions were made in Tris saline and the chemicals, prepared as stock solutions in DMSO, were added to the diluted

143

TABLE II. The Effect of Varying Concentrations of Noncarcinogenic and Carcinogenic Aromatic Hydrocarbons on the Infectivity of HSV-type 2.

Treatment (μg/ml)		Titer of herpes simplex virus (PFU/ml); time in min			Reduction of infectivity at 90 min (%)
		0	45	90	
None		4.2×10^5	2.5×10^5	2.6×10^5	38
DMSO[a]		3.4×10^5	2.4×10^5	2.6×10^5	24
Ant,	100	3.6×10^5	2.6×10^5	2.8×10^5	22
	50	2.8×10^5	2.6×10^5	2.2×10^5	21
	10	2.9×10^5	2.1×10^5	3.3×10^5	0
DMBA,	100	2.3×10^5	1.7×10^5	$<10^4$	>99
	50	2.1×10^5	2.3×10^4	2.1×10^3	99
	10	1.9×10^5	1.3×10^5	6.2×10^4	67

[a] Dimethylsulfoxide was used as the diluent for the chemicals.

TABLE III. The Effect of Temperature on the Inactivation of HSV-type 1 and HSV-type 2 by DMBA.

Virus type and treatment	Temp (°C)	(PFU/ml)		Reduction of infectivity (%)
		0 min	100 min	
HSV-type 1 control	1	4.1×10^6	2.9×10^6	29
	25	4.5×10^6	4.4×10^6	2
	37	4.6×10^6	4.9×10^6	0
+ DMBA[a]	1	3.7×10^6	2.3×10^6	38
	25	3.0×10^6	1.4×10^6	53
	37	3.2×10^6	2.4×10^5	93
HSV-type 2 control	1	2.5×10^5	2.1×10^5	16
	25	1.8×10^5	2.1×10^5	0
	37	2.7×10^5	2.5×10^5	7
+ DMBA[a]	1	1.1×10^5	4.3×10^4	61
	25	1.2×10^5	1.3×10^4	89
	37	1.5×10^5	1.0×10^2	>99

[a] The virus was mixed with 50 μg of DMBA/ml and incubated at 37°, 25°, or at ice bath temperature for 100 min.

virus to give the indicated final concentrations. The test mixtures were sampled following 0-, 45-, and 90-min incubation at 37° and immediately assayed on RK cells as indicated in Materials and Methods.

The data presented in Table II demonstrate the inactivation of HSV infectivity by DMBA at concentrations as low as 10 μg/ml over the 90-min test period. Additionally, a direct relationship was observed between the concentration of DMBA employed and the extent of virus inactivation. Exposure to 1 μg/ml of DMBA did not inactivate HSV after 45 min. In contrast, both Ant, at all concentrations tested, and DMSO were without appreciable effect (over control levels) on the stability of this virus.

Effect of temperature on inactivation of HSV by DMBA. Experiments were conducted to determine whether the inactivation of HSV by DMBA was temperature dependent. In addition, it was decided to study the comparative effect of this chemical on HSV-types 1 and 2. The Seibert strain of HSV-type 1 and the 316D strain of HSV-type 2 were mixed with DMBA, as previously, at a final concentration of 50 μg/ml. Virus controls were diluted in DMBA-free Tris saline. Replicate samples were incubated at 37, 25, and 1° (ice bath). The reaction mixtures were sampled following initial mixing of virus and chemical (0 min) and following incubation for 100 min at the respective temperatures. Samples were immediately titrated in primary RK cultures.

Maximum inactivation of HSV by DMBA occurred at 37° (Table III). Decreased levels of virus inactivation in the presence of DMBA were observed with a reduction in temperature of the reaction mixtures.

Surprisingly, the data in Table III also revealed that HSV-type 2 was more susceptible to inactivation by DMBA than HSV-type 1 at all temperatures tested.

Susceptibility of HSV-type 1 and HSV-type 2 to DMBA. The observation that HSV-type 2 was more susceptible to inactivation by DMBA than HSV-type 1 was investigated

145

TABLE IV. The Effect of DMBA on HSV-type 1 and HSV-type 2.

HSV type	Strain	Treatment	(PFU/ml)		Reduction of infectivity (%)
			0 min	100 min	
1	Hill	Control	7.3×10^5	6.6×10^5	10
		DMBA[a]	7.0×10^5	7.1×10^4	90
1	Haywood	Control	3.0×10^5	4.3×10^5	0
		DMBA	2.3×10^5	2.0×10^4	91
1	Edna	Control	4.2×10^5	4.7×10^5	0
		DMBA	4.2×10^5	5.2×10^4	88
1	Seibert	Control	2.7×10^5	3.2×10^5	0
		DMBA	3.7×10^5	1.4×10^5	62
2	324	Control	1.1×10^4	1.1×10^4	0
		DMBA	1.2×10^4	6.0×10^1	>99
2	198	Control	5.6×10^4	7.7×10^4	0
		DMBA	5.5×10^4	1.0×10^1	>99
2	333	Control	1.0×10^5	9.0×10^4	10
		DMBA	6.0×10^4	7.0×10^1	>99
2	316D	Control	1.2×10^4	1.5×10^4	0
		DMBA	1.4×10^4	7.0×10^1	>99
2	332	Control	1.8×10^4	9.0×10^3	50
		DMBA	1.3×10^4	2.4×10^2	98
2	French	Control	4.2×10^3	5.8×10^3	0
		DMBA	4.3×10^3	$<10^1$	>99
2	186	Control	4.5×10^3	4.8×10^3	0
		DMBA	1.2×10^4	5.0×10^1	>99
2	327	Control	4.9×10^3	4.1×10^3	16
		DMBA	5.6×10^3	5.0×10^1	99
2	307	Control	2.1×10^4	2.0×10^4	5
		DMBA	1.9×10^4	2.0×10^2	99

[a] HSV was mixed with 50 μg of DMBA/ml and incubated at 37° for 100 min.

on a larger scale. The stability of 4 strains of HSV-type 1 and 9 strains of HSV-type 2 to DMBA at a final concentration of 50 μg of DMBA/ml at 37° for 100 min was then established.

The results of this experiment are summarized in Table IV. All 4 strains of HSV-type 1 exhibited a reduction in titer of 91% or less when incubated at 37° with DMBA. All 9 strains of HSV-type 2 tested were inactivated by 98% or more. Control studies revealed the absence of significant inactivation of all viruses by the noncarcinogenic polycyclic aromatic hydrocarbon, Ant (at 50 μg/ml) or DMSO when tested under similar conditions. This data, therefore, points to the selectivity of DMBA for the inactivation of the infectivity of HSV-type 2 as compared to its effect on HSV-type 1.

Discussion. De Maeyer and De Maeyer-Guignard (14) originally reported the inhibition of HSV replication by the polycyclic aromatic hydrocarbon DMBA. Our study of the interaction of herpes simplex virus and polycyclic aromatic hydrocarbons revealed that HSV-type 2 is more sensitive to DMBA than HSV-type 1 as measured by loss of infectivity following direct exposure to the compound. The reaction was a direct *in vitro* effect free of a cell-mediated system and was temperature and concentration (DMBA) dependent. The noncarcinogenic polycyclic aromatic hydrocarbon, anthracene, had no perceptible effect on either of the herpes types.

The polycyclic aromatic hydrocarbons are hydrophobic and lipophilic and have been shown to associate to varying degrees with lipids, proteins, and/or nucleic acids (15–18). The lipid association appears to be less stable than the more stable association of the chemicals with proteins or nucleic acids. As HSV contains all the chemical constituents (19) that the polycyclic aromatic hydrocarbons are known to react with, it is difficult to clearly establish the mechanism of inactivation of HSV by DMBA. A reaction of DMBA at the level of the lipoprotein envelope of HSV could lead to loss of infectivity.

An interaction of chemical and virus at this point might inactivate or alter the overall charge on the virus leading to inhibition of specific attachment mechanisms. The necessity of the virus envelope for attachment and subsequent infection has been questioned, but attachment and penetration appears to be more efficient when the virus is enveloped (20).

The exact serological differences of HSV-type 1 and HSV-type 2 appear to reside in the capsid of the virion (21). These differences in protein makeup could lead to a preferential interaction of DMBA with one and not the other. The specificity of interaction of carcinogenic aromatic hydrocarbons with specific tissue proteins has been shown by Heidelberger and Moldenhauer (16). A specific reaction of DMBA with HSV-type 2 capsid protein could again lead to inactivation or charge alteration and affect viral adsorption, penetration, or uncoating.

The interaction of DMBA with DNA has been extensively studied by several investigators who have found that the reaction of DMBA with DNA is of a low magnitude and appears to be stable and irreversible (17, 18). The DNA of HSV-types 1 and 2 have been shown to differ slightly in density and in guanine plus cytosine content (22, 23). The interaction of DMBA with DNA of HSV could lead to a mutagenic effect of HSV so that it is unable to successfully complete a productive infection. The direct mutagenic effect of DMBA has been shown with bacterial viruses (24), but to our knowledge not with animal viruses. Whether or not the reaction of this carcinogen with a potentially oncogenic virus has a direct effect on the ultimate neoplastic potential of the virus remains to be determined.

Summary. A carcinogenic polycyclic aromatic hydrocarbon, DMBA, was found to inactivate the infectivity of herpes simplex virus type 2 to a greater degree than the infectivity of herpes simplex virus type 1. The reaction was concentration and temperature dependent. The noncarcinogenic polycyclic aromatic hydrocarbon, anthracene, did not affect the infectivity of either type of herpes simplex virus.

1. Pauls, F. P., and Dowdle, W. R., J. Immunol. 98, 941 (1967).

2. Plummer, G., Waner, J. L., Phuangsab, A., and Goodheart, C. R., J. Virol. 5, 51 (1970).

3. Nahmias, A. J., Dowdle, W. R., Naib, Z. M., Highsmith, A., Harwell, R. W., and Josey, W. E., Proc. Soc. Exp. Biol. Med. 127, 1022 (1968).

4. Figueroa, M. E., and Rawls, W. E., J. Gen. Virol. 4, 259 (1969).

5. Epstein, M. A., Achong, B. G., and Barr, Y. M., Lancet 1, 702 (1964).

6. Epstein, M. A., Barr, Y. M., and Achong, B. G., Wistar Inst. Symp. Mongr. 4, 69 (1965).

7. Darlington, R. W., Granoff, A., and Breeze, D. C., Virology 29, 149 (1966).

8. Lunger, P. D., Darlington, R. W., and Granoff, A., Ann. N.Y. Acad. Sci. 126, 289 (1965).

9. Epstein, M. A., Achong, B. G., Churchill, A. E., and Biggs, P. M., J. Natl. Cancer Inst. 41, 805 (1968).

10 Hsiung, G. D., and Kaplow, L. S., J. Virol. 3, 355 (1969).

11. Iwakata, S., and Grace, J. T., N.Y. State J. Med. 64, 2279 (1964)

12. Rawls, W. E., Tompkins, W. A. F., Figueroa, M. E., and Melnick, J. L., Science 161, 1255 (1968).

13. Rapp, F., J. Bacteriol. 86, 985 (1963).

14. De Maeyer, E., and De Maeyer-Guignard, J., Science 146, 650 (1964).

15. Janss, D. H., and Moon, R. C., Cancer Res. 30, 473 (1970).

16. Heidelberger, C., and Moldenhauer, M. G., Cancer Res. 16, 442 (1956).

17. Brookes, P., and Lawley, P. D., Nature (London) 202, 781 (1964).

18. Alfred, L. J., Nature (London) 208, 1339 (1965).

19. Roizman, B., in "The Biochemistry of Viruses" (H. B. Levy, ed.), p. 415. Dekker, New York/London (1969).

20. Darlington, R. W., and Moss, H. L., Progr. Med. Virol. 11, 16 (1969).

21. Wildy, P., and Watson, D. H., Cold Spring Harbor Symp. Quant. Biol. 27, 25 (1962).

22. Goodheart, C. R., Plummer, G., and Waner, J. L., Virology 35, 473 (1968).

23. Plummer, G., Goodheart, C. R., Henson, D., and Bowling, C. P., Virology **39**, 134 (1969).

24. Martin, C. M., Bacteriol. Rev. **28**, 480 (1964).

THERAPEUTICS XIV

By Heather Ashton, E. Frenk and C. J. Stevenson

Herpes Simplex Virus Infections and Idoxuridine

The use of idoxuridine (5-iodo-2′-deoxyuridine, I.D.U.) in herpes simplex keratitis is of proven value although it is only really effective in superficial corneal infections. In a preliminary communication Hall-Smith *et al.* (1962) obtained promising results with the topical application of idoxuridine, 0·1% in aqueous solution or 0·5% in ointment, to cutaneous herpes simplex lesions, but others (Kolzmann, 1963; Burnett and Katz, 1963) had only limited success. However a 0·1% solution of idoxuridine in polyvinyl alcohol with propylene glycol, polyvinyl alcohol and water or polyethylene glycol polysorbate proved more effective than no treatment in 111 patients (Corbett *et al.* 1966). The use of dimethylsulphoxide (DMSO) as a vehicle for the topical application of idoxuridine was reported by Goldman and Kitzmiller (1965). They used 1% idoxuridine in 90% DMSO and 10% distilled water. Seven patients with severe cutaneous herpes simplex infection were treated, with significant improvement and with only slight skin irritation from the solution.

A double blind trial of 5% idoxuridine in DMSO and of DMSO alone was reported by MacCallum and Juel-Jensen (1966). Sixteen patients were in the trial, one of whom defaulted. The comparison was between 21 attacks of facial herpes simplex in this group, 10 of which were treated with idoxuridine in DMSO and the remainder with DMSO alone. The solution was applied to each lesion three times daily for 3 days. The average expected duration of the attack as estimated by the patients when untreated was compared with the average duration in the trial. There was a shortening of the average duration by 6·3 days (64%) for the idoxuridine treated group and 4·1 days (43%) for the dimethylsulphoxide treated group, a difference of 2·6 days between idoxuridine in the solvent and the solution alone. Naseman and Braun-Falco (1970) treating 103 patients with an ointment containing 0·2% I.D.U. and 1·8% DMSO obtained results suggesting that the duration of the infection was shortened. The ointment caused irritation when applied to the genital area and this was diminished by the addition of prednisolone. Genital herpes simplex is a special problem in pregnant women since disseminated herpes simplex of the newborn can be acquired from an infected mother (Hudson and McFarland, 1969).

The efficient treatment of cold sores is important owing to the risk of ocular involvement to the patient and the risk to contacts. There are three situations however when herpes simplex infection can be a more serious problem, namely when recurrent attacks of erythema multiforme ensue, in renal transplant units where immunosuppressive drugs reduce the resistance to infection, and in eczema herpeticum. Topical treatment with idoxuridine in DMSO would seem worth a trial in dealing with milder examples in the first two situations and erythema multiforme can be tolerably well controlled with systemic corticosteroid drugs.

Experience in renal transplant units seems to vary. Spencer and Anderson (1970) noted that of 55 immunosuppressed renal allograft recipients 16 had cold sores. They found that herpes simplex infections appeared more common after transplant than before in those patients subject to recurrent attacks but serious illness with widespread lesions was not seen. Montgomerie and colleagues (1969) described immunosuppressed patients who received renal transplants. In one patient the herpes simplex infection was considered to have caused death and in the other it was an important contributory factor. Three patients used topical idoxuridine in aqueous solution without effect and one of these patients was given systemic idoxuridine. She was a woman aged 30 who had received two cadaveric renal transplants. The dosage of idoxuridine in terms of the body weight is not stated. The patient died and herpes simplex virus was isolated from the oeso-phagus and lungs at necropsy.

The management of eczema herpeticum has been more satisfactory since the availability of systemic antibiotics to deal with pyogenic infection which frequently co-exists with the herpetic infection (Brain, 1950). The early diagnosis of this variety of Kaposi's eruption from that due to vaccinia is important and can be greatly assisted by using immuno-fluorescent antibody techniques such as those of Joseph et al. (1959) and Gardner et al. (1968), where such facilities are available. Death in eczema herpeticum can occur from adrenal necrosis (Brain et al., 1957), from herpes simplex encephalitis (Quilligan and Wilson, 1951), and herpes simplex hepatitis can also occur. Although herpes simplex encephalitis more commonly occurs without skin lesions it carries a high mortality (Olson et al., 1967). A serious illness in a child with eczema herpeticum should arouse suspicion of these complications and suggest the advisability of electroencephalography (Upton and Gumpert, 1970).

When treating a severely ill child with eczema herpeticum the dermatologist may find himself no less experienced in the use of idoxuridine than his colleagues in other disciplines. The decision regarding the use of systemic idoxuridine may arise and can be urgent since response to treatment of herpes simplex meningitis is better if the treatment is given early and since the idoxuridine solution takes time and pains to dispense for intravenous infusion. Nolan and others (1970) used a freshly dissolved solution of 3 G. of idoxuridine powder in 1,000 ml. of 5% glucose in water. The pH was adjusted to 8·2 with dilute sodium hydroxide. Solutions were sterilized by millipore filtration and tested for sterility by inoculation into nutrient broth.

Idoxuridine has been extensively used by Calabresi et al. (1961), who showed that in neoplastic disease, toxic effects were transient and tolerable even when given in doses as high as 620 mg. per kg. body weight. In 8 patients given courses of 400 mg./kg. only 3 had toxic effects and these were minimal. Six patients who had 600 mg. per kg. body weight all had side effects. Nolan and others (1970) used a dosage of 430 mg. per kg. body weight when treating herpes simplex encephalitis. Of the 6 patients treated, all developed stomatitis, loss of hair, thrombocytopaenia and in one case, loss of nails, but all these changes were reversible. Dayan and Lewis (1969) reported cholestatic jaundice in a patient treated with I.D.U., and Silk and Roome (1970) treated a boy aged 6 whose liver function tests showed evidence of liver damage which reversed on recovery. Idoxuridine competes with the utilization of thymidine during the synthesis of deoxyribonucleic acid and therefore the side effects of stomatitis, alopecia and bone marrow depression are to be expected also there must be some risk to the gonads.

Breeden et al. (1966) were the first to report the treatment of herpes simplex virus encephalitis. They treated a male patient aged 34 who had no skin lesions with a total of 550 mg. of idoxuridine per kilogram body weight given by intravenous infusion over 7 days. The patient recovered with no impairment of the mental state but with some neurological sequelae. Some impairment of the liver function was possibly due to the infection and some depression of platelets and granulocytes occurred. Buckley and MacCallum (1967) treated a man aged 41 with idoxuridine; he recovered but with mental and neurological sequelae. Marshall (1967) treated a boy aged 13 with acute neurotizing herpes simplex encephalitis; he made an almost perfect recovery. Evans et al. (1968) treated an 8 year old girl who recovered but with severe intellectual and neurological sequelae. Adams et al. (1969) treated 2 patients who survived and had only transient leucopaenia. Rappel et al. (1969) treated 10 patients with herpes simplex encephalitis with systemic idoxuridine, all of whom recovered with only transient mild toxic effects, but Dayan and Lewis (1969) treated one patient, who had diarrhoea—a side effect of idoxuridine, but died after initial improvement. Adams et al. (1969) treated 2 patients with herpes simplex encephalitis with systemic idoxuridine, both survived and had only transient leucopaenia. Duffy (1969) treated 3 patients, 2 of whom recovered but with neurological sequelae. Silk and Roome (1970) treated a boy aged 6 who recovered but

36

with severe sequelae. Tomlinson and MacCallum (1970) treated 3 patients, all of whom died.

The most encouraging report is from Nolan *et al.* (1970). They reported on 13 patients with herpes simplex encephalitis but the diagnosis was not in all cases confirmed by the finding of herpes simplex virus. Of 7 untreated patients, 3 died, and the 4 survivors had loss of function. Of 6 treated patients 2 died two days before the 5-day course could be completed, the 4 fully treated cases recovered completely.

Review of the literature concerning the treatment of severe herpes simplex virus infections with systemic idoxuridine suggests that side effects, although significant are reversible and, as far as records show, not fatal. Several patients with severe infections have made good recoveries, which are likely to have been due to the drug. Faced with a patient severely ill with herpes simplex virus infection the dermatologist would seem justified in being prepared to use systemic idoxuridine.

REFERENCES

ADAMS, J. H., JENNETT, W. B. and MILLER, J. D. (1969) Drugs Against Viruses. Correspondence. *Lancet*, i, 987.

BIEGELEISEN, J. Z., SCOTT, L. V. and LEWIS, V. (1959) Rapid Diagnosis of Herpes Simplex Virus Infections with Fluorescent Antibody. *Science, N.Y.*, **129**, 640.

BRAIN, R. T., DUDGEON, J. A. and PHILPOTT, M. G. (1950) Kaposi's Variecelliform Eruption. *Br. J. Derm.*, **62**, 203.

BRAIN, R. T., PUGH, R. C. B. and DUDGEON, J. A. (1957) Adrenal Necrosis in Generalized Herpes Simplex. *Archs Dis. Childh.*, **32**, 120.

BREEDEN, C. J., HALL, T. C. and TYLER, H. R. (1966) Herpes Simplex Encephalitis Treated with Systemic 5-iodo-2-deoxyuridine. *Ann. intern. Med.*, **65**, 1050.

BUCKLEY, T. F. and MACCALLUM, F. O. (1967) Herpes Simplex Virus Encephalitis Treated with Idoxuridine. *Br. med. J.*, ii, 419.

BURNETT, J. W. and KATZ, S. L. (1963) Study of use of 5-iodo-2'-deoxyridine in Cutaneous Herpes Simplex. *J. invest. Derm.*, **40**, 7.

CALABRESI, P., CARDOSO, S. S., FINCH, S. C., KLIGERMAN, M. M., VON ESSEN, C. F., CHU, M. Y. and WELCH, A. D. (1961) Initial Clinical Studies with 5-iodo-2'-deoxyuridine. *Cancer Res.*, **21**, 550.

CORBETT, M. B., SIDELL, C. M. and ZIMMERMAN, M. (1966) Idoxuridine in the Treatment of Cutaneous Herpes Simplex. *J. Am. med. Ass.*, **196**, 441.

DAYAN, A. D. and LEWIS, P. D. (1969) Idoxuridine and Jaundice. Correspondence. *Lancet*, ii, 1073.

DUFFY, G. J. J. (1969) Herpes Simplex Encephalitis—Neurological Implications and Treatment. *J. Neurol. Neurosurg. Psychiat.*, **32**, 634.

EVANS, A. D., GRAY, O. P., MILLER, M. H., VERRIER JONES, E. R., WEEKS, R. D. and WELLS, C. E. C. (1967) Herpes Simplex Encephalitis Treated with Intravenous Idoxuridine. *Br. med. J.*, ii, 407.

GARDNER, P. S., McQUILLIN, J., BLACK, M. M. and RICHARDSON, J. (1968) Rapid Diagnosis of Herpes Virus Hominis Infections in Superficial Lesions by Immunofluorescent Antibody Techniques. *Br. med. J.*, iv, 89.

GOLDMAN, L. and KITZMILLER, K. W. (1965) Topical 5-iodo-2'-deoxyuridine in Dimethylsulphoxide (DMSO): New Treatment for Severe Herpes Simplex. *Ohio St. med. J.*, **61**, 532.

HALL-SMITH, S. P., CORRIGAN, M. J. and GILKES, M. J. (1962) Treatment of Herpes Simplex with 5-iodo-2'-deoxyuridine. *Br. med. J.*, ii, 1515.

HOLZMAN, H. (1963) Zur Herpes simplex Therapie in der Dermatologie mit 5-jod-2'-desoxyuridin. *Z. Haut-u. GeschlKrankh.*, **35**, 86.

HUDSON, A. W. and McFARLAND, C. (1969) Disseminated Herpes Simplex in a Newborn. A Consequence of Infection in the Mother. *J. Am. med. Ass.*, **208**, 859.

MACCALLUM, F. O. and JEUL-JENSEN, B. E. (1966) Herpes Simplex Virus Infection in Man Treated with Idoxuridine in Dimethyl Sulphoxide. Results of Double-Blind Controlled Trial. *Br. med. J.*, ii, 805.

MARSHALL, W. J. S. (1967) Herpes Simplex Encephalitis Treated with Idoxuridine and External Decompression. *Lancet*, ii, 579.

MONTGOMERIE, J. Z., BECROFT, D. M. O., CROXSON, M. C., DOAK, P. B. and NORTH, J. D. K. (1969) Herpes-Simplex-Virus Infection after Renal Transplantation. *Lancet*, ii, 867.

NASEMANN, TH. and BRAUN-FALCO, Q. (1970) Virustatische Substanzen in der Lokalbehandlung herpetischer Dermatosen. *Therapie. Gegenw.*, **109**, 222.

NOLAN, D. C., CARRUTHERS, M. M. and LERNER, A. M. (1970) *Herpesvirus Hominis* Encephalitis in Michigan. Report of Thirteen Cases, including six Treated with Idoxuridine. *New Engl. J. Med.*, **282**, 10.

OLSON, L. C., BUESCHER, E. L., ARTENSTEIN, M. S. and PARKMAN, P. D. (1967) Herpesvirus Infections of the Human Central Nervous System. *New Engl. J. Med.*, **277**, 1271.

QUILLIGAN, J. J. and WILSON, J. L. (1951) Fatal Herpes Simplex Infection in a Newborn Infant. *J. Lab. clin. Med.*, **38**, 742.

RAPPEL, M. (1969) Drugs Against Viruses. *Lancet*, ii, 272.

SILK, B. R. and ROOME, A. P. C. H. (1970) Herpes Encephalitis Treated with Intravenous Idoxyridine. *Lancet*, i, 411.

SPENCER, E. S., ANDERSEN, H. K. (1970) Clinically Evident, Non-terminal Infections with Herpesviruses and the Wart Virus in Immunosuppressed Renal Allograft Recipients. *Br. med. J.*, iii, 251.

TOMLINSON, A. H. and MACCALLUM, F. O. (1970) The Effects of Iodo-deoxyuridine in Herpes Simplex Virus Encephalitis in Animals and Man. *Ann. N.Y. Acad. Sci.*

UPTON, A. and GUMPERT, J. (1970) Electroencephalography in the Diagnosis of Herpes-Simplex Encephalitis. *Lancet*, i, 650.

AUTHOR INDEX

Albert, Daniel M., 9
Ashton, Heather, 151

Barahana, H.H., 110

Capps, Worth I., 24

Derge, Jefferey D., 86
Dinter, Z., 42
Docherty, John J., 140

Ellery, B.W., 120

Frenk, E., 151

Gainer, Joseph H., 24
Goldberg, Robert J., 140
Gwaltney, Jack M., Jr., 17

Hampar, Berge, 86
Hill, Paul, 24
Howes, D.W., 120

Kabuta, Hidefumi, 61
Klingeborn, B., 42

Larkin, Edward P., 50
Long, Jack, Jr., 24
Lytle, C.D., 128

Martos, Lidia M., 86
Melendez, L.V., 110

Nakagawa, Yoh, 61
Nichol, F.R., 98

Peeler, James T., 50

Rabson, Alan S., 9
Rapp, Fred, 140
Read, Ralston B., Jr., 50

Stevenson, C.J., 151
Sullivan, Robert, 50

Tierney, John T., 50

Ulbrich, A.P., 136
Underwood, G.E., 98

Walker, John L., 86

Yamamoto, Shigeru, 61